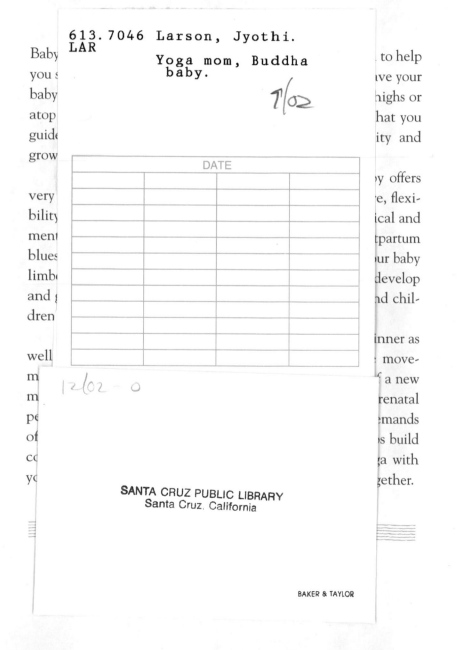

Baby ... to help you s ... ve your baby ... highs or atop ... hat you guide ... ity and grow ...

very ... y offers ... e, flexibility ... ical and ment ... tpartum blues ... ur baby limb ... develop and g ... d children ...

well ... inner as m ... e movem ... f a new m ... renatal pe ... emands of ... s build c ... ga with y ... gether.

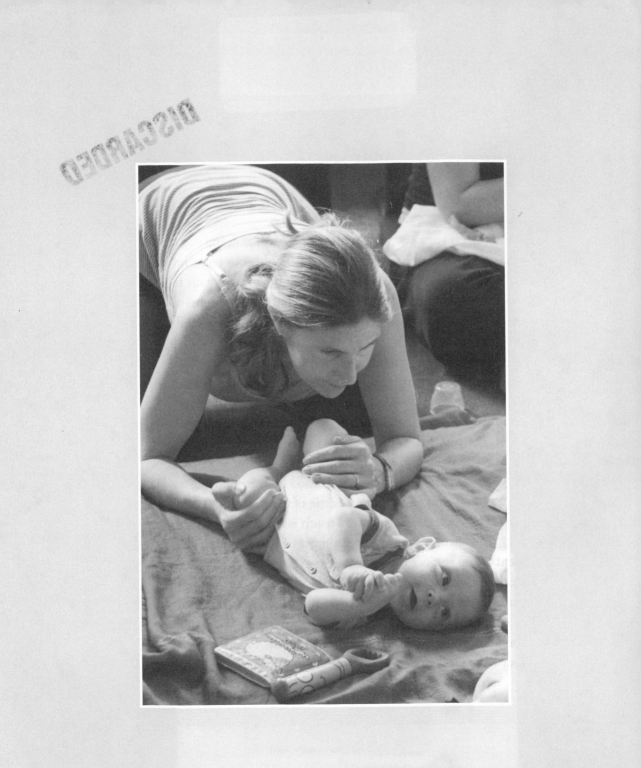

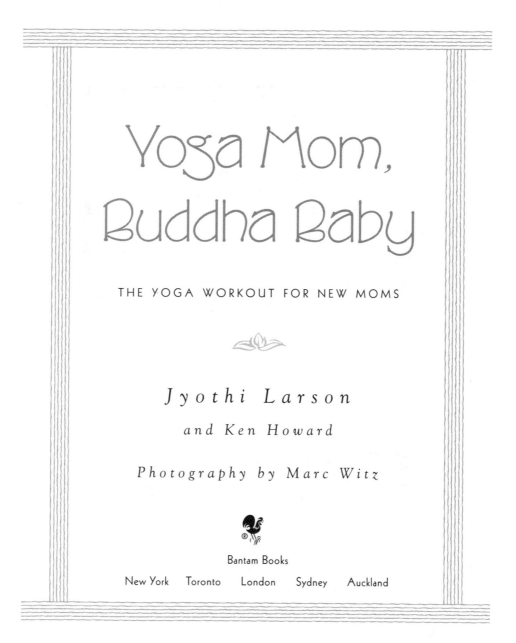

Yoga Mom, Buddha Baby

THE YOGA WORKOUT FOR NEW MOMS

Jyothi Larson

and *Ken Howard*

Photography by Marc Witz

Bantam Books

New York Toronto London Sydney Auckland

YOGA MOM, BUDDHA BABY

PUBLISHING HISTORY
Bantam trade paperback / April 2002

Book design by Ellen Cipriano

Library of Congress Cataloging-in-Publication Data
Larson, Jyothi.
Yoga mom, Buddha baby : the yoga workout for new moms /
Jyothi Larson and Ken Howard; photography by Marc Witz.
p.   cm.
Includes index.
ISBN 0-553-38093-1
1. Motherhood. 2. Yoga, Haòha. 3. Exercise for women.
4. Mothers—Health and hygiene. 5. Postnatal care.
I. Howard, Ken (Kenneth) II. Title.
RG801 .L37 2002
613.7'046'082—dc21
2001043791

Published simultaneously in the United States and Canada

Bantam Books are published by Bantam Books, a division of Random
House, Inc. Its trademark, consisting of the words "Bantam Books"
and the portrayal of a rooster, is Registered in U.S. Patent and
Trademark Office and in other countries. Marca Registrada. Bantam
Books, 1540 Broadway, New York, New York 10036.

PRINTED IN THE UNITED STATES OF AMERICA
RRH   10 9 8 7 6 5 4 3 2 1

Dedicated to my Yoga Mom
Bella
and my Buddha Babies
Rachel and Mikela

Acknowledgments

From the bottom of my heart, thank you to all the beautiful moms and babies who have come to my classes and who continue to grace my life. You have inspired me and taught me so much.

Thank you to all the Yoga Moms and Buddha Babies who appear in this book:

Yoga Moms and Buddha Babies:

Natasha and Uma
Danielle and Van
Nanette and Jasmine
Stacy and Hannah
Min and Daniel
Francesca and Brando
Trisha and Aimee
Sylvia and Hannah
Adele and Luciana
Laura and Natalie
Liz and Jasper
Marcia and Maya
Darcy and Rupert

Yoga Moms-to-be:
Anne-Marie Cooleen
Cathy Q. Bailey
Fay Savage
Sharmila Seth

Thank you to Natasha and Uma for all those beautiful boat poses. Thank you to Marc Witz for taking these gorgeous photos and bringing the spirit of yoga to the page. Thanks to sue.p. and Valerie Clayman Pye for making sure we looked our best. A heartfelt thank you to Glen Edelstein for his skill in bringing it all together—and remember to work those abs. My thanks also to Healing Works for their generosity in sharing studio space for the class photos.

Thank you to Ken Howard, my co-author, who turned the classes I love to teach into a book. And a special thanks to my wonderful editor Robin Michaelson—your expert guidance and enthusiasm have made this an amazing book.

—JL

Thank you to my wife Jessica for her patience and invaluable editing; my family, for their love and support; and in particular my Grandma Connie, for inviting me along to her yoga class when I was eight years old. Thanks also to my co-author Jyothi Larson, who expanded my appreciation of what yoga can bring to life, and to our editor Robin Michaelson, whose detailed attention gave shape to the book.

—KH

Contents

Foreword

Welcome, Yoga Moms!

Congratulations on becoming a parent! And hello, babies: welcome to this world.

Babies are transformative—whether this is your first child or second or fifth, your life will never be the same again. Every new life changes us. Managing that change, and growing along with it, occurs on many different levels—emotional, physical and spiritual. I hope you will allow yoga to enter your life and help enhance the change your new baby brings.

Yoga that you do along with your child—with your child in your arms, on your tummy, resting against your thighs or sleeping peacefully at your side—is powerful in the way that it connects the changes in your body with your new child. You grow together, every week and every day. Your baby continually reveals new abilities. And the same is true with how your body changes after birth—hormones cycle through, pounds are shed while strains are shifted. The weight is no longer centered in your pelvis; instead your shoulders, neck and arms are taxed as you feed your baby, hold her and carry her around.

Along with the physical challenges of motherhood comes the joy of just touching and bonding with your baby. This all becomes part of the yoga routine. Babies find the touch comforting, and it's a wonderful opportunity to stretch, strengthen, relax and meditate with your baby. You have your whole life to do yoga by yourself; take advantage of the special time in your child's early life by doing yoga with her.

I have been practicing yoga for over twenty-five years, and I am grateful for how it has helped me through the transitions and challenges that my life is continually providing. My mother practiced yoga, and I saw the great difference it made in her life—she felt more fit, and it also helped her to relax and reduce stress. So I was compelled to check it out. I started taking classes when I was a teenager, and fell in love with the practice. The postures made me feel strong and toned. Yoga also awakened my spirituality; I began to understand the body-mind connection and to pay more attention to how I connected with society. Over the years, I have studied with different teachers and at various schools. The style of yoga that I practice and teach is something I call "Eclectic Yoga." It is a combination of techniques and teachings I learned at different schools and from different teachers. I tend to use what speaks to me and what works for me.

I moved to New York City to study fashion design. After working in the field for five years and having my first daughter, Rachel, I was drawn to a different calling—full-time yoga! I made the switch because I believed I should have a purpose in my vocation, and for me that wasn't designing clothes; it was practicing yoga and teaching it to others. I became certified through the Integral Yoga Institute in New York City and began teaching.

My postpartum classes were born out of my own feelings as a new mother. I cried every afternoon at three o'clock for weeks after Rachel's birth. I suffered from feelings of isolation (winter can be so long!) and questions such as "Will I ever get out of the house?" It made no sense to me: I had this beautiful, healthy baby. Why was I crying? I was also questioning whether I would ever feel good again about my body. Based on my playtime with Rachel and my love of yoga, I started developing ways to do yoga with my baby. I wanted to share this with other mothers. We could get stronger and more fit as our babies grew. New mothers' bodies did not have to ache; by being aware of posture and by stretching and strengthening, women could really help themselves recover from the stress of pregnancy, delivery and being a parent.

The postpartum techniques I developed also came out of the success of my prenatal classes. I loved my moms and felt I was deserting them at a very important time in their lives by not giving them anywhere to come to after the birth of their babies. They needed a special place to do yoga geared for their postpregnancy bodies that was also built around the excitement and demands of the beautiful new beings in their lives. It has been exciting over the years to see more and more yoga classes for moms and babies, moms and children and now "Daddy and Me" classes coming into existence.

My own children—Rachel and Mikela—were avid yogis for years and still do some yoga with me. However, Rachel, now eleven years old, doesn't think yoga is very "cool." Mikela, age seven, still does some yoga with me, often jumping on me and making me aware of my strength and our closeness. Motherhood continues to be a challenge, though in different ways, and I'm thankful for the strength yoga has helped me to develop.

On other personal levels, yoga has helped me with the demands of motherhood as well as with divorce and the loss of loved ones. Yoga has helped me find joy and peace. Yoga will help you become more in tune with your feelings and your intuition—striking a balance between what's best for you, your baby and your family. Besides giving you an understanding of your body, yoga will give you strength and self-esteem.

I am renewed every time new mothers and their babies come to class. This is a singular time in life as women experience motherhood for the first time. It is a privilege for me to be a witness to this again and again. This time is special not only for first-time moms, but for any mom, as subsequent births place different demands. These first few months of creating a mother-child bond are precious, and it's enlightening and exciting for me to play a part in this for many women.

Even if you have doubts—"I'm so out of shape"; "Will I be able to do this?"; "I'm not flexible"—let your ego go. Whatever shape you're in, whatever flexibility you have or do not have, you are in the perfect place to practice yoga.

A few months ago, a mother and her three-month-old daughter came to my class through the invitation of another mom. She asked to just watch, because, as she explained, "I'm out of shape and my baby hardly lets me put her down, and I don't know how this will work." She and her daughter ended up participating fully in the class. Afterward, she said she felt happy and excited that she could actually do something for her continual lower back-ache and would definitely return. The rewards of yoga with your baby can be wonderful.

Over the years I have watched friends discover yoga and have seen the changes it makes in their lives. My hope is that this book will bring that joy to women and their babies beyond those I reach through my classes. Yoga is a simple but deeply enriching way to take care of yourself and expand your bond with your child. It lets you stretch and meditate as you touch and hold her, and to begin working with her growing body to keep her limber, healthy and strong. In this book, I have shared the most important lessons that I teach in my classes. It is your introduction and guide. And if you are already taking a class, the book will offer a reinforcement of proper technique and, I hope, new ways to practice your yoga.

Congratulations on your new role. This is a time of growth for you and your baby and your new family. I hope yoga adds to that experience and becomes a part of the rest of your life.

Jyothi Larson
New York City

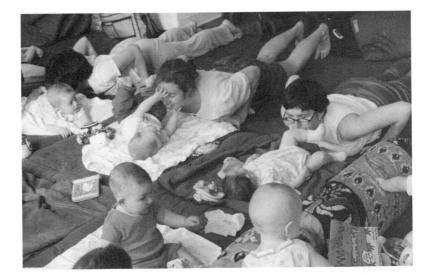

Yoga Mom, Buddha Baby

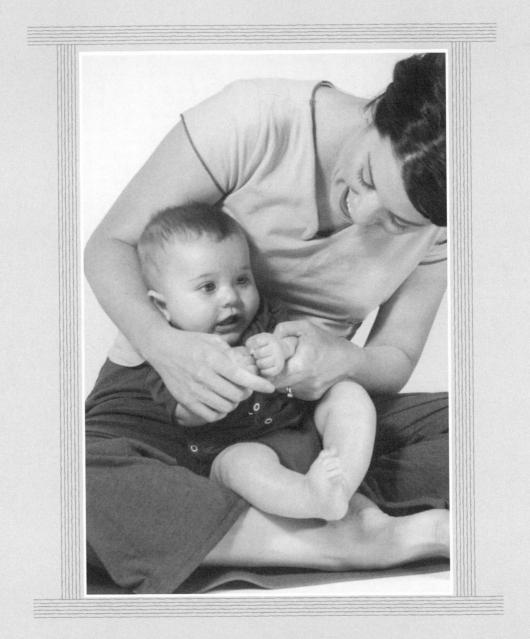

One

Introduction to Yoga for New Moms

What Is Yoga?

The word "yoga" means "yoke" in Sanskrit—a joining, a oneness. When people think of yoga they usually think of the physical aspect, but yoga was first practiced as meditation, a striving of the individual to become one with the universe. Two texts in particular are important in yoga: the ancient Indian epic the *Mahabharata* and the *Yoga Sutras* by Patanjali. Both teach how to live a "yogic life": what to eat, how to practice yoga, how to control the mind and how to sustain one's yoga practice and reach for an ever-broader level of consciousness.

The main goal of yoga is to find the peace and joy of who we are. This place is known as the *anandamayakosha* or bliss body (peaceful, calm, truth). One gets to this place through practicing asanas (postures), breathing, relaxation, and meditation.

Yoga is very important to me and is a big part of my life. Yes, I still get stressed from life—raising children, dealing with finances, keeping my home, work and life going. But my practice gives me a way to get grounded and remain in touch with the

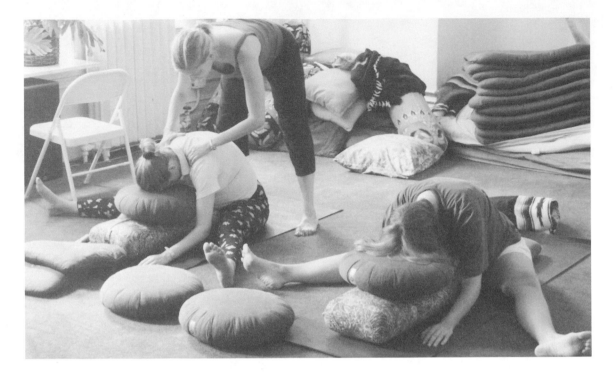

things in life I find very important: my growth and spirituality, my children, family and friends.

Yoga is constant development. You learn what your body can do as well as the body-mind connection. Through focused breathing and meditation, I have expanded my understanding of myself and my interaction with the world.

Yoga is an open-minded practice that says there is not one way to get to the truth. Yoga gives me a philosophy: some days I feel I understand many things, other times nothing. That's life; that's yoga. It's a philosophy that we work toward, learning at our own rate. The message that I take from this is to find the peace and joy of who I am and who we are.

Why Baby Yoga?

Baby yoga is yoga practiced with your baby. It is doing yoga to help you stretch, relax and strengthen as you hold your baby, have your baby next to you or have your baby leaning against your thighs or atop your belly. Baby yoga is also special yoga positions that you guide your baby through to encourage natural flexibility and growth. Baby yoga takes advantage of babies' love of being touched. They are getting used to and exploring a new environment, and touch is both reassuring to them and a way to connect to the world. And, of course, moms love to touch their babies.

For you as the mom, practicing yoga with your baby offers very tangible physical results: it helps improve your posture, flexibility, strength and endurance. It contributes to your physical and mental well-being and can help to ward off potential postpartum blues.

A happier, calmer, stronger mom makes for a happier, calmer, stronger baby. The exercises will help your baby limber up, sleep easier and relax and will encourage his muscles to develop and grow. Many babies are also calmed or entertained by the chanting and children's songs that go along with some of the postures.

The "Eclectic Yoga" that I teach is meant for the beginner as well as someone who has been practicing for years. The movements I use respect the special demands put on the body of a new mother. Exercise builds strength and flexibility during the prenatal period. After the baby is born, a mother is addressing the demands of nursing, cradling and carrying a growing baby. Yoga helps build confidence and a strong and healthy body. Practicing yoga with your baby is a wonderful way to add joy to your first year together.

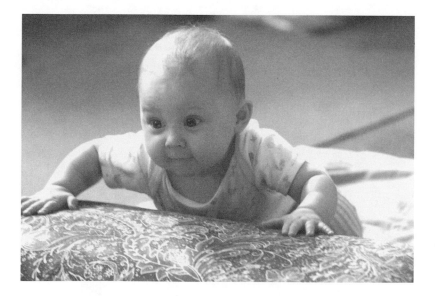

This Is Your Book

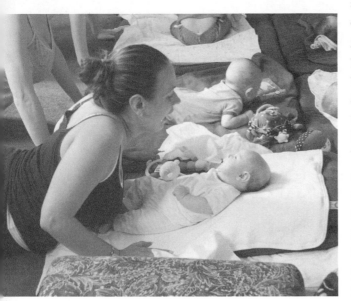

I have worked with hundreds of women and their babies in the classes that I teach. Many have asked for pointers and tips before and after class, and this book is an extension of those requests. The book is intended as a guide and companion, designed to help you practice whatever approach to yoga is comfortable for you. I have included "beginner" series that help any mother, regardless of fitness level or yoga experience, get the great benefits of the postures and movements. There are also more advanced positions and suggested sets to stimulate the most dedicated yogi. And there is everything in between, including a ten-minute routine that can help energize you in the morning or in the middle of the day and relaxation postures to be done before bed to help you get a good night's sleep.

Buddha Babies

"Buddha Baby" is my term for a healthy, content baby. I often feel as I hold newborns and babies and look into their eyes that this is about as close as one can get to the divine energy. As mothers, we are our child's "first guru." But our babies and children are also great teachers to us. Yoga done with your baby builds nonverbal lines of communication and enhances the special joy of sharing your baby's discovery of his new life.

Partner Parents

Yoga Mom, Buddha Baby

It is wonderful to do yoga together as a family, and I have provided positions that a partner can do with you and your baby. Parenting is also about communication, and partners are encouraged to join in the breathing and relaxation exercises, which offer a nonverbal way to be together as a family.

A Time for Yoga

While it would be ideal to be able to set aside up to an hour or more during the day to practice yoga, I recognize that ten minutes in your busy day may be all that you can dedicate to yoga, and that's okay too. This book contains short practices in addition to longer series, and I encourage you to do your favorite stretch whenever you feel inclined. You may also want to get together with other new moms: form a yoga group, or if there is a class in the area, go once or twice a week. Many yoga studios are now offering "Mommy and Me" and sometimes "Daddy and Me" classes.

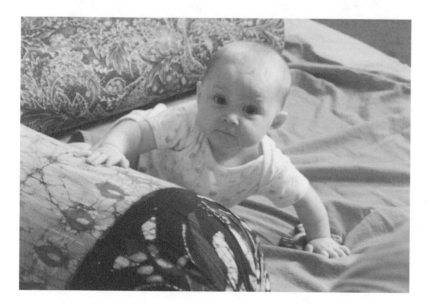

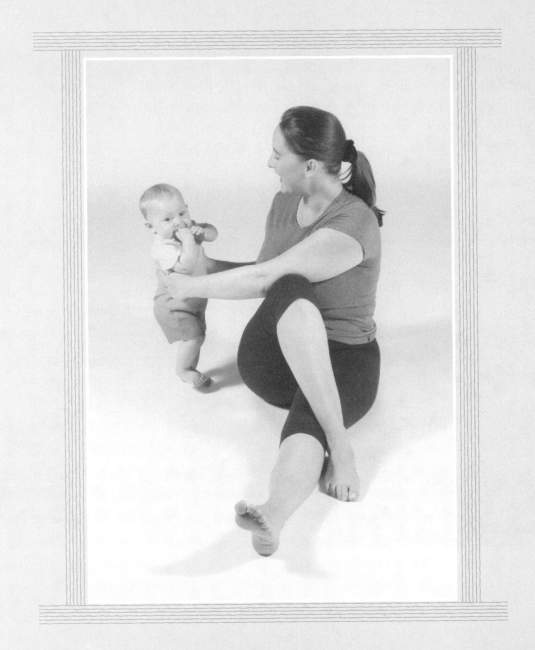

Two

Covering
the Basics

≈⟐≈

Practicing Yoga with Your Baby

Remember that "yoga" means "to join." It unites mind, body and breathing through asanas, or poses, to bring strength, flexibility and calm to the mind and body. It requires very little—not much space, very little "equipment" and just as much time as you can give it (though more is better)—and the returns are significant. You will feel calmer, stronger, more flexible and more in control of your life and body after practicing yoga for just a short period of time.

When your baby arrives, the asanas will help you get back in shape and maintain your body while allowing you to build a bond with your child. As your body changes, the positions change, from beginning asanas you can start right after delivery to more challenging positions as you grow stronger (you will need to keep up with the lifting, carrying and stroller-pushing of your growing baby!). The relaxation poses help you sleep at night and stay calm during the day.

The asanas are for your baby too as she develops from being able to roll over and hold up her head to crawling. Your baby is not only at your side as you do yoga but also rides on your belly and thighs, is held to your chest and lifted up and down, getting kissed and doing her own mommy-assisted asanas. Movement for your baby becomes incorporated into your asana practice. Very quickly you will see your baby do her own beautiful cobras. In one of the classes I taught, a year-old toddler named India often fell asleep sucking her toe—talk about flexibility! Babies are natural yoginis.

Getting Started

The book is organized into twelve chapters. The first six chapters introduce the basics of baby yoga and breathing exercises, relaxation poses and warm-up postures you will use throughout the book. Chapter Seven gives future moms a head start with prenatal yoga. The next several chapters follow your baby's growth: Chapter Eight, the first six weeks; Chapter Nine, the next six weeks; and Chapter Ten, up to one year. Chapter Eleven offers special routines for focused yoga—waking up in the morning, a quick stretch, a targeted routine to help you relax and a ten-minute series for a fast but satisfying session. Chapter Twelve has postures your partner can do with you and your baby. The Afterword gives some ideas for continuing your and your baby's yoga practice as your baby moves into toddlerhood and beyond.

Each chapter describes asanas to help you stretch, strengthen and bring balance to your body and life. While some of the asanas focus on mom and some focus on baby, all are meant to be done with baby at mom's side (if not actually participating). This doesn't mean mothers shouldn't do yoga by themselves; maybe someone else is taking care of the baby, or maybe she is sleeping (finally!) and you're in the mood to do some yoga. But having your baby involved makes a very special addition and enhances your yoga practice—and, as you will see, babies love it!

Each chapter has, in addition to the asanas—which can be done separately for a quick stretch or together in a series—suggested routines. These series of asanas give you a total body workout. You can add your favorite asanas to the suggested routine or mix and match, depending on your body's needs and how much time you have. The chapters also include special postures moms can guide their babies through to encourage flexibility, good health and joy.

Noted within specific asanas in the book are any medical cautions, such as avoiding or modifying a pose if you have had a C-section or are experiencing specific physical problems. It is important, however, to check with your doctor before beginning any exercise, including yoga, both while you are pregnant and after you have delivered your child.

What You Will Need

Wear loose, comfortable clothing. It is better not to wear socks—there is less chance that your feet will slip—but wear them if your feet are cold. If you will be wearing them, try to find socks with non-skid bottoms. You will also need:

- A Blanket
- A Pillow
- A Yoga mat (same as "sticky" mat)
- A Strap (optional)
- A Cushion from a couch or chair (optional)
- A Bolster (optional)
- An Eye pillow (optional)
- Music (optional)

Yoga mats, straps, bolsters and eye pillows are available at many health clubs, sports stores and yoga studios.

What Your Baby Will Need

Dress your baby in comfortable clothes appropriate to the season and the temperature in the room.

To Begin

Find a warm, comfortable, quiet room with enough space that you can lie down with your hands and feet fully extended. A rug can be useful, though you may still want to lay a towel or mat over it for added cushioning. If you are on a bare floor, make sure to use a sticky mat. Make a comfortable spot next to yourself for your baby. She can be on a towel or on her own blanket or mat.

As you do your yoga, keep in mind the basics—proceed gently, never force a movement and remember to breathe! You'll be terrific.

Yoga Talk

Here are definitions to help you with some terms and phrases I use throughout the book:

ASANA: A movement or posture.

INHALE/EXHALE: The focused taking in and letting out of breath. Your breath is coordinated with the movements in an asana.

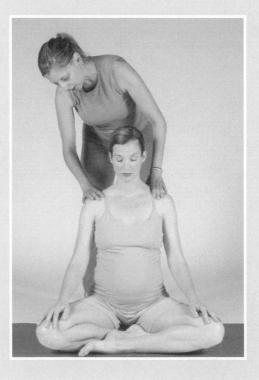

LENGTHENING UP THROUGH THE SPINE: This describes sitting in proper posture. As you sit and lengthen your spine, focus on feeling energy move up from the base of your spine, following the natural curves, and rise to the base of your skull and out through the top of your head (crown); feel as though you are sitting a little taller, not slouching.

SITTING/"SITS BONES": It is important when sitting for meditation or certain asanas that your spine is lengthened, with your spine and the top of your head (crown) reaching for the sky (or "up toward the heavens") and your sits bones—the bones at the bottom of the pelvis—anchored and moving down into the floor (or "down toward the earth"), grounding you.

OPEN UP THE CHEST: This phrase describes how you free your chest of tightness. Your shoulders are relaxed. Your shoulder blades are back a little and sit on top of your ribs. Feel your whole heart center open.

BRING YOUR BELLY BUTTON TOWARD YOUR SPINE AND LIFT UP: This phrase is used to help you focus on the movement of your abdominal muscles in toward your spine, providing important muscle support for various positions. However, it does not mean pulling your muscles in so much that you can't breathe—make sure you are comfortable.

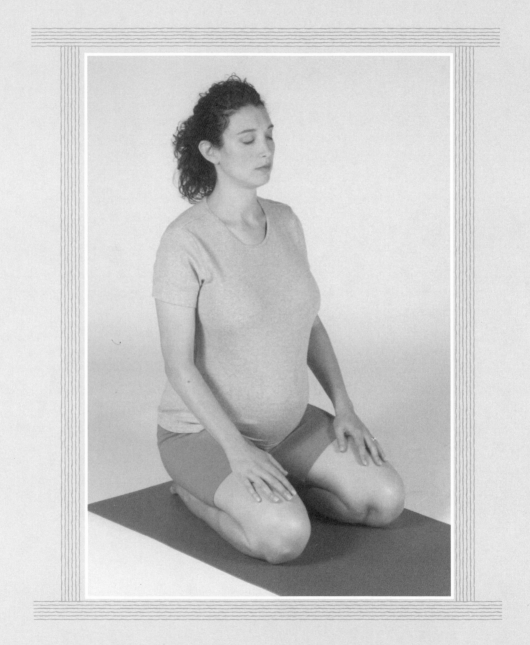

Three

Breathe!

Breathe:
To bring more oxygen into your
lungs and bloodstream
To introduce calm to your body
To quiet your thoughts
To center yourself
To renew and revitalize

Most of the time you don't think about your breathing, it just happens. An important aspect of yoga is watching your breath and feeling how you breathe, focusing on how the breath feels coming into your body and how your muscles work to bring breath in and let it out. "Yogic breathing" can bring with it a center of calm in the middle of chaos, a source of energy that also offers "mindfulness," a place you bring yourself to appreciate the moment. This can be especially important for you as a new mother; suddenly your life is filled with another being, and that can be totally overwhelming. While having a baby is unbelievably fulfilling, at times you can feel as though you have lost part of yourself. Mindfulness is a way to get back to who you are.

Yoga breathing also creates vitality, bringing more oxygen into your lungs and bloodstream to feed your cells and give you *prana*, or new energy. You will feel rejuvenated and healthful. It will help

Mindfulness

Mindfulness is the art of being present. It is not thinking about or analyzing the past or thinking about the future. For me, it is about breathing. Just be where you are, whether it is lying, sitting or walking. Start to watch your breath. Feel the inhalations ("Three-Part Breath") and the exhalations. When your mind focuses on the breath, everything else falls away.

Don't stress out over how long your inhalation or exhalation is. Let it be natural.

Moms ask me: "Am I doing it right?" Yes: breathe, watch your breath, "just be" and you are doing it right.

calm you during pregnancy and help you focus and relax your body during labor. And once you have delivered, it will allow you to breathe away stress and breathe in energy and serenity.

Yoga offers different methods of breathing for different needs and contexts. Some are wonderful for rejuvenation, others for calming; still others provide a deep serenity to accompany meditation. You will probably find that you favor some over others, and at different times some will be preferable to others. To decide which to do, just listen to how your body feels!

What Does It Mean to Listen to Your Body?

"Listening to your body" is being in tune with it and responding to what it is telling you. Body wisdom tells us when a position is uncomfortable, when a certain yoga posture or *pranayana* (breathing practice) shouldn't be done or even when a particular pose is just the thing to relieve tension. These are important messages anytime in our lives, but they are particularly important during

Yoga Mom,
Buddha Baby

14

the body changes associated with pregnancy and early mother-hood.

A good way to listen to the body is by going to each part of the body and seeing or listening to what it is feeling. Once you feel a tightness or an ache or pain, you can do something about it. For instance, achy necks and shoulders can be common for new mothers. What can you do to ease these aches?

- Ask yourself: "How am I holding my baby?"
- Change your posture. When the neck and shoulders ache, do a pose to relieve these aches.
- When you are in a yoga position, how does it feel? Where are you feeling the stretch? If it feels too intense, ease up on the stretch.
- As you breathe, feel and watch your breath, concentrating on its coming into your lungs, feeling it in the belly and experiencing how your lungs feel as they expand and what it feels like to expand your chest even farther to let in more breath.
- Bring awareness to different parts of your body: your toes, legs, pelvis, spine, arms, abdomen, shoulders, neck and head. Inside your body, become more aware of the muscles, organs and joints.
- Trust your intuition and your instincts. If something doesn't feel right, do not continue the position, or perhaps hold it for a shorter time than recommended.
- Your body knows what is best for you. During pregnancy, listen to aches and pains by responding with stretches and movement. During labor, use your breathing to help your body deliver your baby. And after delivery, when you are caring for your new baby, again pay attention to the needs of your body and incorporate breathing, stretches and exercise to answer those needs.

Be open to what you're feeling; accept it. In our society, we tend to want to push, push, push to do more. Listen to what your body is telling you. Sometimes doing less is doing more.

Breathe!

Tailor Sitting

We are all so used to sitting in chairs, but how many of us are still comfortable sitting on the floor? Tailor sitting—named for how tailors used to sit and stitch—means sitting on the floor in a comfortable cross-legged position. This is so good for you!

If you need support, sit with your back against a wall (or back-to-back with a partner). You can put the soles of your feet together, stretch your legs out, or you can sit with your ankles crossed; pick whichever position is most comfortable. And that may vary, depending on how your body feels today. You may also find it more comfortable to sit on the edge of a pillow or blanket under your sits bones.

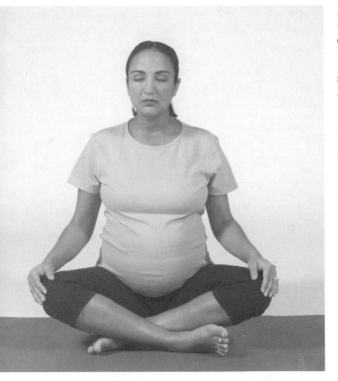

Press your sits bones—the bones at the bottom of your pelvis—down into the floor or blanket. Bring your hands to your knees and relax your shoulders. Feel the support of the floor. Bring your awareness to your tailbone, then your lower back (sacrum). Start lengthening up through each vertebra, feeling yourself getting a little taller. Continue to lift your vertebrae up through your neck and to the base of your skull. Move your head from side to side and shoulder to shoulder a little bit, finding your center. Then keep lengthening up through the spine. Open up your chest by bringing your shoulders back so the shoulder blades feel as if they are sitting on your ribs. Let your shoulders relax. Think about the pelvis and lower body connecting with the earth—the pull of gravity—and the upper body lengthening and reaching up to the heavens.

Breathing moves you through all the yoga postures, so it is important to become conscious of it. When you are stressed, breathing tends to become shallower; when you are relaxed, it becomes deeper. Practice your breathing so that you can slow it down and take deeper breaths to reach a more restful state. Conscious breathing will also prepare you for labor by helping you to work with your contractions and to vocalize along with your breathing as a natural and healthy way to focus your energy during delivery.

Belly Breathing

Belly breathing tones abdominal muscles as well as teaching you how to breathe fully and consciously. This is important because some people have shallow breathing, others tense breathing. Breathing can be relaxed in a smooth rhythm. This is the way your baby will breathe. When your baby is born watch her relaxed, rhythmic breathing; the belly fills up on the inhalation and gets smaller on the exhalation.

To begin: In your tailor sitting position, bring your awareness down to your belly and your baby. Inhale through your nose and feel as well as visualize your belly expanding with breath. Exhale, feeling your belly button move back toward your baby, as if your abdominal muscles are "hugging" the baby. Inhale again and feel your belly getting bigger with breath. Exhale, feeling your belly button coming toward your baby.

Belly check: Be aware of proper posture. Don't slouch as your breasts become heavier; it's important to open up through your chest. Ground your sits bones into the floor. Be comfortable with the breath.

Repetitions: Begin with two to three minutes of belly breathing, focusing on your abdominal muscles, then continue for as long as you like before starting your practice.

Yoga taught me to just keep breathing, which was helpful during labor when emotionally you want to shut down. Yoga allowed me to not get in the way of what was happening, the body opening itself; it knows what to do.

—LAURIE AND SON JACK

Breathe!

17

Three-Part Breath
(Deergha Swaasam)

This breathing brings calmness into the body. It increases energy and vitality by bringing more oxygen into the lungs. Deergha Swaasam also helps turn your awareness to the abdominal muscles as you concentrate on breathing in and out.

This type of breathing can be practiced whenever you feel a need to center yourself. It is also an excellent way to relax and focus before beginning postures.

To begin: This breathing practice is divided into three parts to best fill the lungs completely. It is easiest to learn Deergha Swaasam by starting out comfortably seated or lying down on your side.

Part one: Breathe in through your nose, and feel and visualize your belly getting bigger, expanding outward. It is almost as if you are releasing your abdomen up. Exhale and feel your belly button move back toward your spine, your abdomen contracting in.

Part two: Inhale again, feeling your belly, lower back, and rib cage expand. Exhale, feeling your rib cage, lower back, and belly button condense back toward your baby.

Part three: Inhale again, bringing breath into your belly and lower back, your rib cage, middle back, then chest and upper back. Exhale, feeling your chest and rib cage condense and your belly button come back toward your baby.

Belly check: If you feel light-headed, return to your regular breathing.

Cleansing Breath with
Movement

This breathing practice is great for helping to relieve tension. You can also do this sitting, without movement.

To begin: Start in a standing position. Inhale through your nostrils and then exhale through an open mouth with the sound of ahhhh!

When I was in labor the breathing I had practiced was very helpful; I did a cleansing breath and it got me through the 25 hours of labor, it got me through each contraction.

—SHARON AND DAUGHTER ORA
AND SON EVAN

*Yoga Mom,
Buddha Baby*

Inhale and bring your breath into your belly, your rib cage and then your chest. As you inhale, bring your arms overhead. Exhale with sound, sending out breath from your chest, your back and then your rib cage (your rib cage will contract). Your belly will get a little smaller; you are "hugging your baby" with your abdominal muscles. Your arms come down as you exhale; bend your knees. You can even visualize the breath leaving through the pelvic floor. This will focus you on the connection between your breathing and muscle control. Being aware of the connection will help you work with the contractions during labor.

Belly check: Relax and let go. The ahhh sound is on the exhale, and you will make many sounds as you deliver your baby. During Rachel's birth, my midwife told me I was making too much noise and she couldn't concentrate, but I didn't care; I went on making the sounds I wanted to!

Repetitions: Three times. Practice whenever you feel the need.

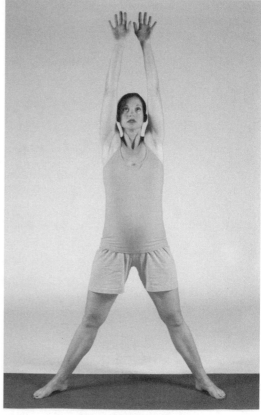

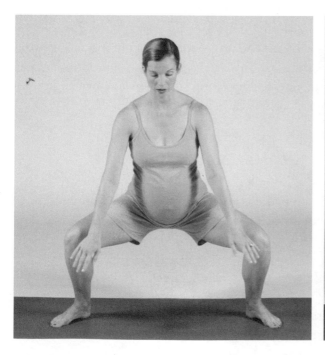

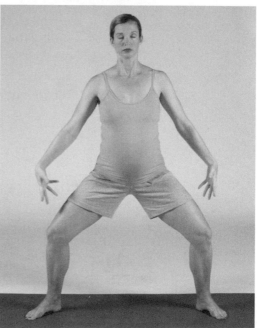

Proper Posture

It is important for you to be aware of your posture throughout your yoga practice; it is necessary for proper breathing and alignment and general well-being. During pregnancy, you'll notice how your center of gravity shifts as your weight increases and your body changes. Once you have delivered, you'll experience another change in your posture and balance, as your breasts change and you lose weight put on during pregnancy.

After Birth

Parts of your body—your belly, breasts, buttocks and internal organs—will change during the weeks following labor. Focusing on your breathing will sensitize you to what's happening all over your body. The breathing will also help to center you during a time when your hormones are fluctuating and when you may be anxious over your new responsibilities as a mother.

Belly Breathing

Belly breathing strengthens abdominal muscles and brings focus to the mind. Practicing belly breathing also balances mind, body and soul.

Where's Baby: In your arms or on a blanket in front of you

To begin: Starting in a comfortable seated position, bring your awareness down to your belly. Inhale through your nose and feel as

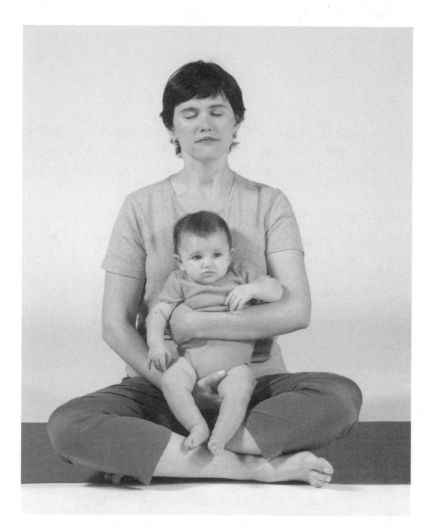

well as visualize your belly expanding with breath. Exhale, feeling your belly button move back and up toward your spine. When you are first doing belly breathing, you might want to put your hands on your belly to feel it expand with the inhalations and condense with exhalations.

Body check: Be aware of proper posture. Be careful not to slump forward; keep your chest open. Ground your sits bones into the floor.

Repetitions: Begin with two to three minutes of breathing, focusing on your abdominal muscles, then do this as long as you like.

Breathe!

Three-Part Breath
(Deergha Swaasam)

This breathing practice calms the body and increases energy and vitality by bringing more oxygen into the lungs. Deergha Swaasam also helps bring your awareness to the abdominal muscles as you concentrate on breathing in and out.

If your baby is agitated, pick him up and begin Deergha Swaasam, breathing with your baby. As you time your breathing to your baby's, or bring calm to your breathing, he may also begin to relax.

This type of breathing can be practiced all the time, whenever you feel a need to center yourself. Whenever I feel anxious or overwhelmed I remember to breathe like this and I immediately feel better. It is particularly nice to practice this breathing while feeding or holding your baby. The baby picks up the calmness and positive feeling.

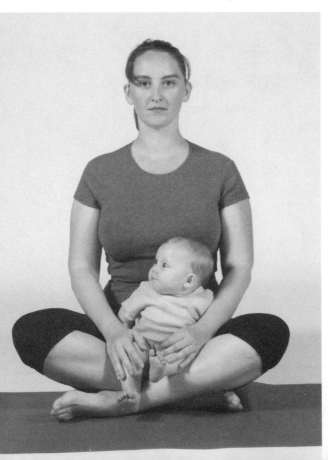

Where's Baby: Held against your chest

To begin: This breathing practice is divided into three parts to best fill the lungs completely (it will enable you to take seven times as much oxygen into your lungs). It is easiest to learn Deergha Swaasam by starting out comfortably seated or lying down.

Part one: Breathe in through your nose, and feel and visualize your belly getting bigger, expanding outward. It is almost as if you are releasing your abdomen up. Exhale and feel your belly button move back toward your spine, your abdomen contracting in.

Part two: Inhale again, feeling your belly, lower back and rib cage expand. Exhale, feeling your rib cage and lower back condense and your belly button move back toward your spine.

Part three: Inhale again, bringing breath into your belly and lower back, your rib cage, middle back, then chest and upper back. Exhale, feeling your chest and rib cage condense and your belly button move back toward your spine.

Just to show you where your lungs are: put your fingers right above the collarbones. When you inhale, you'll feel the collarbone rise—that's how high up your lungs go!

Body check: If you feel light-headed, return to your regular breathing.

Cleansing Breath with Movement

This breathing practice is terrific for releasing tension. You can add movement at any time. Yawning during these breathing practices is normal; your body is experiencing the benefits of bringing more oxygen in and it wants even more, so you yawn!

Where's Baby: On a blanket in front of you. She will enjoy watching you.

To begin: Stand with your legs open slightly more than hip width apart. Inhale through your nose with your mouth closed, taking a nice deep inhalation. Lift your arms over your head. You may want to bring your palms together in a prayer position or simply stretch each hand toward the sky; see which way is most enjoyable for you. Exhale through your open mouth, sighing as you let the air out—ahhhh! As you exhale, bend your knees and drop your arms down, making contact with your baby.

Body check: Relax and let go.

Repetitions: Do the cleansing breath with movement three times, then stand for a few minutes noticing how you feel.

Breathe!

Alternate Nostril Breathing (Nadi Sudhi)

Alternate nostril breathing balances the right and left sides of your body. In Eastern philosophy, the right side is male, the sun and "yin"; the left side is female, the moon and "yang." By alternating breaths through each nostril, you focus energy on both sides, bringing balance to the body.

Where's Baby: Sitting in your lap or lying in front of you

To begin: Make a fist with your right hand and then release your thumb and ring and pinky fingers. Use your thumb to close off the right nostril. Inhale slowly through the left nostril. When the lungs are full, close your left nostril with your ring and pinky fingers, release your thumb, and exhale through your right nostril. Your head, neck and spine should be aligned, with your chest open. Keep your elbows relaxed. Inhale through the right nostril, close off the right nostril with your thumb. Release your ring and pinky fingers, and exhale through the left nostril. Continue this pattern of exhaling and inhaling for up to three minutes. Breathe

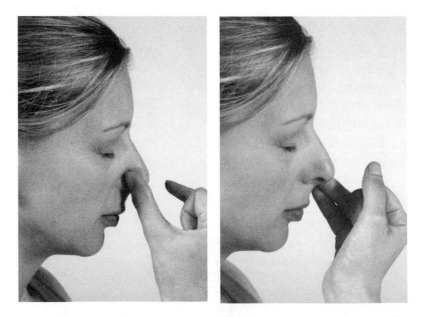

in and out slowly and deeply while keeping your entire body relaxed. On the inhalation try counting to sixteen and on the exhalation to eight.

Body check: Check your posture. As you become acquainted with this breathing, let the inhalation be longer than the exhalation.

Repetitions: Five to ten minutes

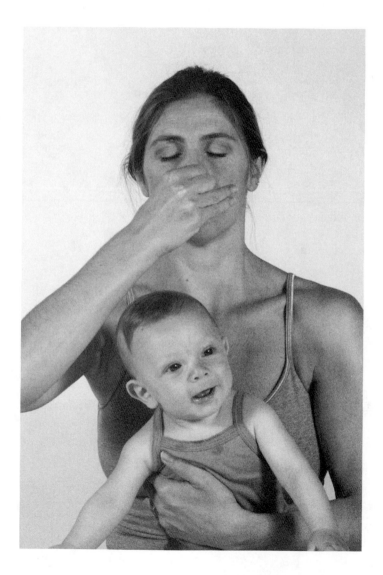

Kapaalabhaati
(Deep Diaphragm Breathing)

This warming, energetic breath tones the abdominal muscles and gives the internal organs a massage. You can begin this breathing practice right after birth but not with a forceful exhalation. After six weeks, your exhalation can increase in force. Babies are entertained by this practice.

Once you learn the breathing, you can use it anytime; it's a lifelong habit. When I get frazzled and realize I am holding my breath because I am tense, I breathe and bring in more oxygen.

—ELIZABETH AND SON
ALEXANDER

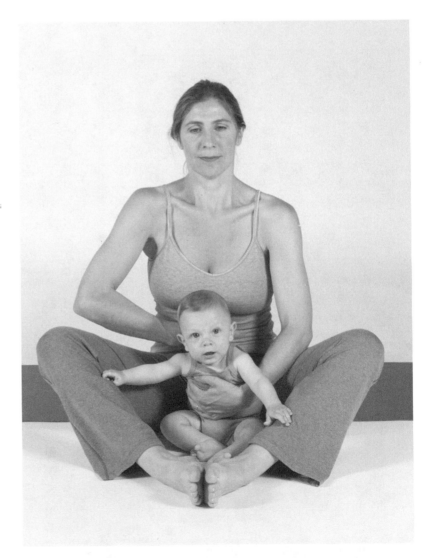

*Yoga Mom,
Buddha Baby*

Medical caution: Never do this breathing during pregnancy.

Where's Baby: On a blanket in front of you or held in your arms against your chest

To begin: This breathing practice focuses on the exhalation/inhalation cycle using the abdominal muscles. The technique is divided into several rapid, forceful exhalations—emptying the lungs of air by snapping the abdomen in. As you exhale, the belly comes in and the inhalation happens naturally on its own.

Begin the first round of exhalations by pulling in your abdomen in a rapid series, so it's like your diaphragm is making you blow your nose. If you are not sure which way your abdomen is going, put your hand on your abdomen to check that the muscles are moving in as the air is being pushed out. Try pulling your abdomen in ten quick times. On the last exhalation, empty your lungs completely.

Now take in a nice deep inhalation and exhaling begin another round of kapaalabhaati. This time do fifteen exhalations and for the third round do twenty exhalations.

Body check: Check your posture. Let your breathing be steady and comfortable. Make sure to take in a nice deep inhalation and exhalation between each round.

Repetitions: Three rounds, working up to twenty breaths each round

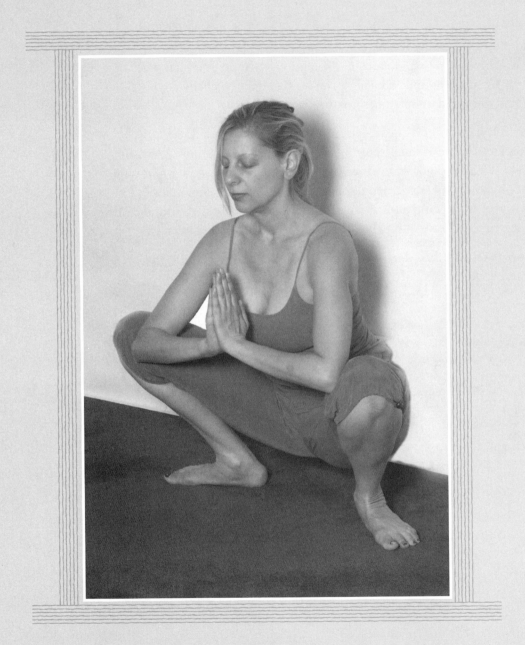

Relax and Meditate

Relax:
To reduce tension
To allow the body to
revitalize and rejuvenate
To help the body and mind
prepare for labor and delivery
To relax throughout your life

We live in a wonderful and amazing but also crazy and stressed world. Many of us believe that the more we do, the better. It is common to hear someone say, "I'm exhausted." Giving the body time to relax is a way to rejuvenate, to recharge and to de-stress.

For a new mother, it can be difficult to find any time to relax, especially if you have other children. It would be great to take twenty minutes a day for relaxation, but even five or ten minutes will reap benefits.

As you relax, watch your breath and see what comes into the mind. Then let that thought fall to the side, or go from the thought back to the breath so you do not get caught up in it. When you return to just watching the breath, thoughts leave and you return to the present. Breathing and relaxation work together. As you inhale, visualize yourself filling with peace and calmness. As you exhale, see yourself releasing tension.

Meditation is nondoing; it is just being. We always feel as if we have to be doing something. To just sit and be still and watch your breath and allow yourself to be quiet provides calmness and puts things in perspective. It allows not only our body to relax, but also our mind and spirit.

Relax and Meditate

Relaxation Poses to Do While Pregnant

Relaxation allows the body and mind to become still and peaceful. These positions also help with sleeping, which can become difficult during pregnancy.

Whichever position you are lying in, feel your body at ease, totally supported by the blankets, pillows and floor beneath you. See if you can feel as though there is no part of your body that you need to hold on to. Surrender; let go. Begin to watch your breath. As you inhale, watch your breath move into your entire body, and then feel your awareness reach your baby, communicating with him. "Listen" to your baby to see what he may want to share with you. Babies are very aware and present in your womb. See your baby surrounded by a beautiful light and watch as this circle grows, getting larger until you too are encircled in the light. Let the breath flow on its own. Now envision a stream of warm golden relaxation right above your head. Feel it as it starts moving into every part of your body. Your baby feels this relaxation, as does every bone, muscle, organ, nerve and cell of your body. Stay in this relaxation state for ten minutes. To come out, return your awareness to your breathing. As your breathing deepens, feel *prana*, fresh energy, in every part of your body. Slowly wiggle your toes and fingers and stretch out your legs and arms.

Reclining Buddha

This comfortable, relaxing position is just about letting go.

Props: Cushion, pillow or blanket

To begin: Lie on your left side. Bend your right leg, with the right knee on the floor. Bring your left arm behind you and your right arm in front. Place a nearby cushion or blanket under your head and one under the right knee; you may also want one under your right elbow. Allow your body to relax.

Belly check: Be comfortable.

Length: Ten minutes

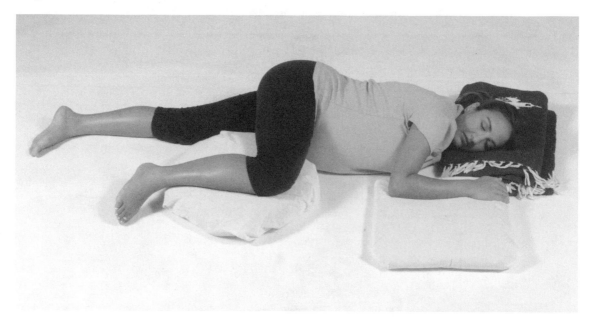

Supported Bound Angle
(Supta Baddha Konasana)

This is a terrific position for quick rejuvenation. The pose opens up the chest, as well as the hip and groin area, encouraging blood flow. It also helps alleviate backaches.

Medical cautions: Do not do this posture if you have any nerve problems in your neck or spinal disk conditions.

Props: Cushion or bolster, blankets, optional strap and eye pillow

To begin: Sitting, bring the soles of your feet together. If you are using a strap, place it around your feet as in the photo. You can also place pillows under your knees. Bring the bolster or cushion against your lower back and place blankets on the bolster. Hold the bolster as you lower yourself onto it. Place a rolled towel or blanket under your neck. Use an eye pillow if you'd like. Let your arms rest away from you on the floor, your palms turned skyward.

Belly check: Relax and breathe.

Length: Five to ten minutes

Being tense or under strain is part of early parenthood. But you realize you can relax, that there is a way to relax with your child; sometimes it is relaxation on the floor and sometimes doing a walking meditation with your baby. Relaxation exercises give you the skill to take five or ten minutes to make quiet time for yourself.

—ELIZABETH AND
SON ALEXANDER

Yoga Mom,
Buddha Baby

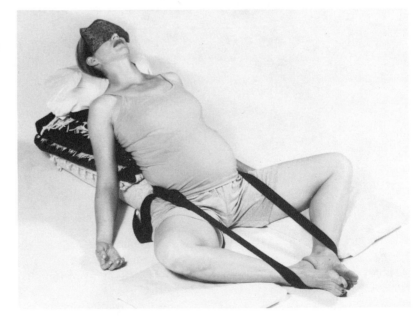

Side Lying Position

This is a position you are already spending a lot of time in!

Props: Cushion, pillow or blanket

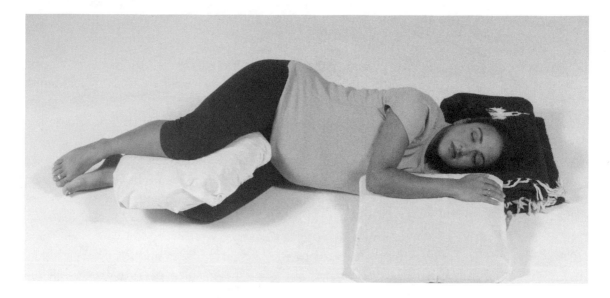

To begin: Sit on the floor with a blanket, rug or mat underneath you, and gently lower yourself down to a position lying on your side, your knees bent. It is recommended that you lie on your left side; however, you already have so many restrictions that if you would like to lie on your right side, that's okay. Place a blanket or cushion underneath your head and position a rolled-up blanket or cushion between your knees. Take another cushion or folded blanket and rest your arm on top of it. Close your eyes and relax into the position, letting tension melt from your body. Get to a place where you can let go, feeling as though there is no part of your body that you need to hold on to. With each exhalation, let yourself melt down into the floor a little farther.

Belly check: Make sure there is no strain on any part of your body. Add or adjust the cushions or blankets for maximum comfort.

Length: As long as you want

Relax and Meditate

Restorative/Relaxation Poses to Do After Your Baby Is Born

I learned how to relax. When I'm pushing a stroller, waiting for the subway, sitting down and breast-feeding, I'm relaxing, and she feels that.

—ELKE AND DAUGHTER SORCHE

These poses allow the whole body to relax—the body isn't being asked to do anything. They bring calmness to the body and mind, which is vitally important because caring for a new baby can be exhausting. Your getting in tune with yourself and becoming less stressed is something your baby will pick up on.

Each pose offers a unique way to relax and rejuvenate. Try different ones on different days, depending on how you feel. These are great to do if you have ten minutes on your own; you can also do them with your baby on your chest.

Whichever relaxation pose you are in, feel your body relax, totally supported by the blankets, pillows and floor beneath you. See if you can feel as though there is no part of your body that you need to hold on to. Surrender; let go. Begin to watch your breath. As you inhale, watch your breath move into your entire body. As you exhale, let go. Envision a stream of warm golden relaxation right above your head. Feel it as it starts moving into every part of your body, every bone, muscle, organ, nerve and cell. Stay in this relaxation state for ten minutes. To come out, return your awareness to your breathing. As your breathing deepens, feel *prana*, fresh energy, in every part of your body. Slowly wiggle your toes and fingers and stretch out your legs and arms.

Savasana

Savasana is known as the corpse pose. This posture helps bring deep relaxation to your entire body while quieting the mind. It is a good position to do with three-part breath. Traditionally savasana is done without props under the body, but I recommend using blankets or bolsters, as they give support to the lower back and cervical spine (neck).

Yoga Mom,
Buddha Baby

34

Props: Cushion, blanket or bolster

To begin: Lie down on your back, with a cushion or bolster tucked under your bent knees. Place a small rolled-up blanket under your neck and put a blanket over yourself for warmth, if needed. Breathe fluidly and let your mind and body relax.

Body check: Make any adjustments in your position to make yourself comfortable.

Length: Ten minutes

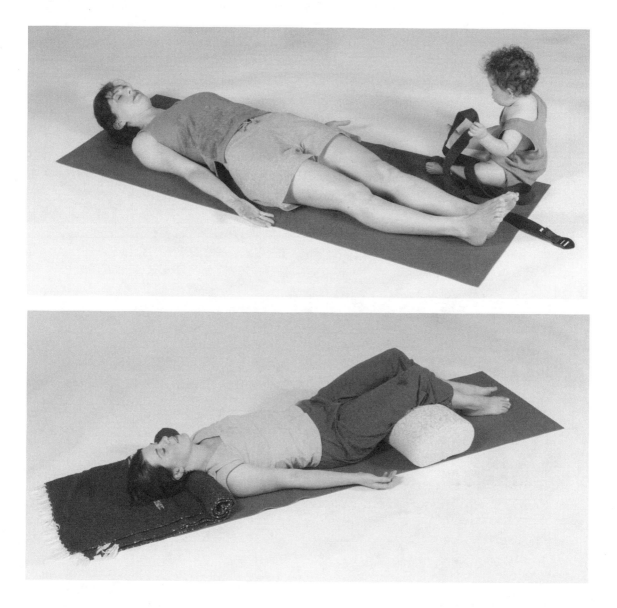

Supported Reclining Pose

This very calming position opens up the chest and helps respiration.

Props: Cushion, pillow or blanket

Where's Baby: On a blanket beside you or against your chest

To begin: Lie down on your back on the floor or a bed, placing a cushion between the floor (bed) and your back; position the cushion under your chest area and parallel to your spine. Position your head and chest slightly higher than your abdomen, pelvis and legs. Let your arms extend away from you, palms facing the sky.

Body check: Make any adjustments in your position to make yourself comfortable. Try two rolled blankets under your knees—it feels good.

Length: Ten minutes

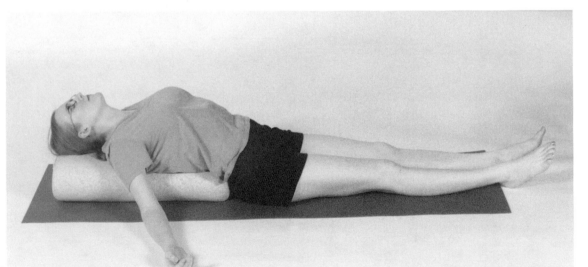

Yoga Mom,
Buddha Baby

Om Chanting

The sound "om" is known as the universal sound of creation. Also called the healing vibration, it reaches different levels of energy as it is generated and moves through your body. It is very soothing and focusing. When you are used to doing it, you feel serenity and a great feeling of harmony with your surroundings.

To begin: Sit in a comfortable, upright position. Take in a nice deep inhalation. Exhale with your mouth open and make an OOOOOOH sound; this is the first part of om. Bring your lips together and hum "mmmmm." Feel the vibration in your throat and lips and then feel it move down into your chest and back, your ribs, your belly and your lower back, finally letting the sound finish at the base of your spine. Begin your second om by inhaling once again. After three oms, sit quietly and feel the vibration in your body.

Belly check: If you feel light-headed, focus on the pelvis's reaching down into the ground or discontinue chanting.

If you are following your om with meditation, you can begin to intone "so hum," which means "I am that." Inhale on "so" and exhale on "hum."

Jack loves when I chant om; his eyes go wide. Maybe he remembers it from in utero—it is a very resonating sound.

—LAURIE AND SON JACK

When Stella gets agitated, the sound of the om helps her relax; it is something different coming into her world.

—JODY AND DAUGHTER STELLA

Prenatal

Women have told me that chanting om during labor has really helped them.
When to do it: Before meditation, and anytime you want to relax and center yourself.

After Birth

When to do it: Before meditation, and anytime you want to relax and center yourself. It is also beneficial to do when your baby is agitated.

Where's Baby: Sit your baby on your lap or hold her as you chant (you can walk and chant at the same time). Direct the vibrations from the oms from your body to your baby's body. The sound will often soothe a cranky baby.

Supported Bound Angle (Supta Baddha Konasana)

This is a terrific position for quick rejuvenation. The pose opens the hip and groin area, encouraging blood flow. It also helps alleviate backaches. It opens up the chest and is great for new moms because they can get really slumped forward with all the feeding, carrying and holding of their baby.

Medical cautions: Do not do if you have any nerve problems in your neck or spinal disk conditions.

Props: Cushion or bolster, blankets

Where's Baby: You can put your baby right on your chest or have your baby close by.

To begin: Sitting, bring the soles of your feet together. You can also place pillows under your knees. Bring the bolster or cushion

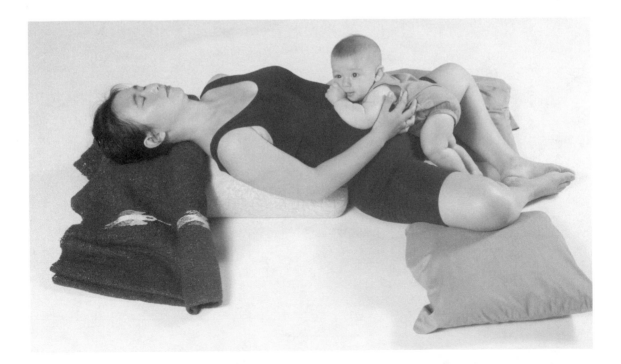

against your lower back; you can also place blankets on the bolster if you'd like. Hold the bolster as you lower yourself onto it. Place a rolled towel or blanket under your neck. Let your arms rest away from you on the floor, your palms turned skyward. If your baby is on your chest, wrap your arms around her.

Body check: Relax and breathe.

Length: Five minutes

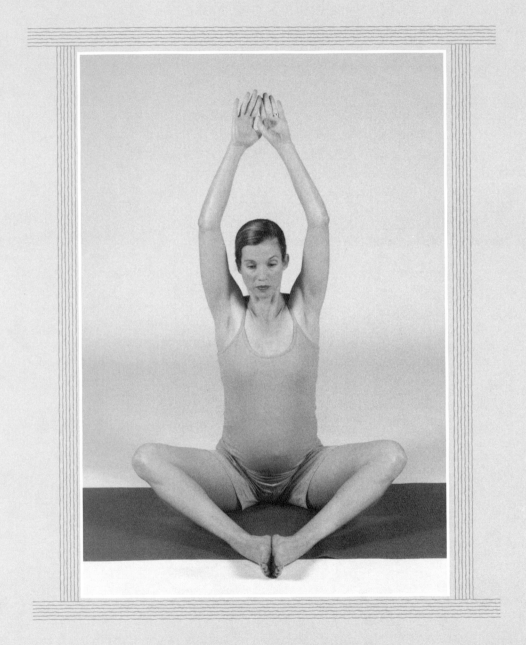

Five

Warm Up and
S-T-R-E-T-C-H

❧

> Stretch:
> To warm, lengthen and
> relax muscles
> To bring calmness and focus
> to your thoughts
> To build entire-body flexibility
> To calm aches and pains
> To experience renewal of
> body and mind

❧

Warming up requires focusing your breathing and energy on the "here and now," checking your posture and where your shoulders are, lining up your vertebrae in a sitting or standing position and letting go of your tension and worries. You are then in a proper mind to begin gentle movements to warm your muscles and joints as a lead-in to additional asanas. Each routine starts out with a warm-up exercise. Many of these are done holding your baby.

Warm-ups incorporate stretches. Stretching is important because every muscle set in the body—in the legs, back, arms, neck and everywhere else—exists as a pair of antagonistic muscles. When one muscle lengthens, its opposite contracts. As we go about our daily lives—walking up stairs, holding our babies, preparing food, exercising, even just sitting—we often overuse one muscle group, stressing that set so it lengthens, while its complementary muscle contracts . . . and contracts . . . and contracts, until it is a tight ball deprived of oxygen, causing pain, decreasing mobility and interfering with blood circulation. Stretching warms and lengthens muscles, allowing them to relax and freeing you from tightness and pain.

Stretching contributes to maintenance of your overall body

balance. You'll have more of a need for this as your body changes during pregnancy and after delivery. Stretching lengthens over-used muscles, such as those in the back that can be strained from the added weight to your shoulders and arms as you hold and feed your baby. When muscles are overused, they are less effective, and they can also be sore and pull the skeletal system out of alignment. Periodic stretching can alleviate the misalignment, and regular stretching can help avoid it altogether.

Prenatal

Warm-up stretches relieve tension in different parts of the body. You can do one or two sets whenever you need them.

Half Neck Rolls

Half neck rolls relieve tension in the neck and shoulders. I do these many times a day.

To begin: Inhale. As you exhale, lower your chin down toward your chest. Take three deep breaths. Notice what you feel in the back of your neck. Inhale and bring your head back up to center. Exhale and bring your right ear toward your right shoulder. Take three breaths. Inhale and slowly raise your head back to center. Exhale slowly and repeat to the left side. Now put the movements together. Inhale, and as you exhale, lower your chin to your chest. Inhale, bringing your right ear up to the right shoulder. Exhale, moving your chin down to your chest. Inhale, bringing your left ear up to your left shoulder. Exhale, moving your chin down to your chest, then bring your head back to center.

Do neck rolls slowly, with one breath flowing into the next. Be aware of what you are feeling in your neck and shoulders.

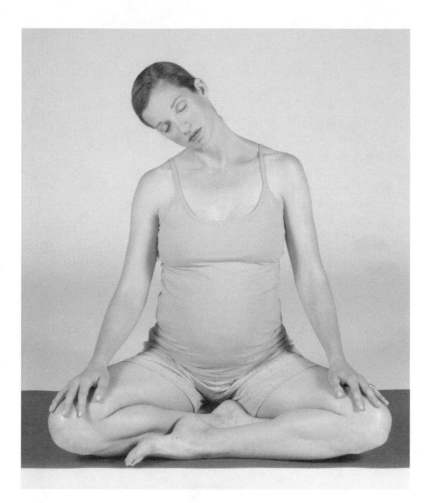

Belly check: Be aware of your posture. As you do the neck rolls make sure your jaw is relaxed; check by opening your mouth and moving it from side to side and up and down. Let your shoulders relax as well.

Repetitions: Three times on each side

Shoulder Rolls

Shoulder rolls open up the chest and upper back and relieve tension in the shoulders. They are excellent for stress relief. This movement also helps relieve the "turtle back" posture that many people have.

To begin: Rest the fingertips of each hand on the respective shoulder, thumb toward the back. As you inhale, bring your elbows forward and lift them toward the ceiling; feel your back opening up. Exhale and bring your elbows back behind you and down; feel your chest opening. Make three circles. Repeat three times in the opposite direction.

Belly check: Be aware of your posture. If you are sitting, make sure that your back is lengthened and your sits bones are anchored to the floor. If you are standing, check your alignment.

Repetitions: Three circles in each direction

After being in the same position for a while—like holding a colicky baby, nursing, sitting in a bad position—it can stress the lower back. Now I do poses to get things aligned and give myself flexibility.

— JODY AND DAUGHTER STELLA

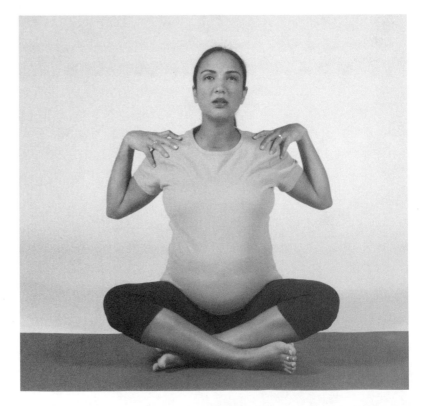

Yoga Mom,
Buddha Baby

After Birth

When you hold and feed your baby, even when you look down at her because she is so beautiful, you tighten your neck and shoulder muscles, putting strain on your entire body. It's nice to do warm-up stretches after feeding your baby or carrying her around. You can also stretch while you hold your baby in the grocery line, in an elevator, wherever.

Half Neck Rolls

Bigger breasts, breast-feeding, bottle-feeding and carrying a baby can add tension to the back and neck muscles. Half neck rolls relieve tension in the neck and shoulders.

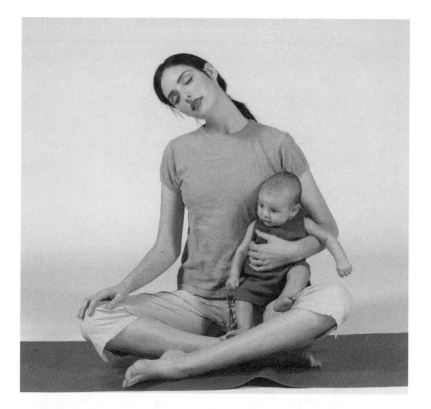

Where's Baby: Your baby can either be in your arms or lying next to you.

To begin: Inhale. As you exhale, lower your chin down toward your chest. Take three deep breaths. Notice what you feel in the back of your neck. Inhale again and bring your head back up to center. Exhale and bring your right ear toward your right shoulder. Take three breaths. Inhale and slowly raise your head back to center. Exhale slowly and repeat to the left side. Now put the movements together. Inhale, and as you exhale, lower your chin to your chest. Inhale, bringing your right ear up to the right shoulder. Exhale, moving your chin down to your chest. Inhale, bringing your left ear up to your left shoulder. Exhale, moving your chin down to your chest.

Do neck rolls slowly, with one breath flowing into the next. Be aware of what you are feeling in your neck and shoulders.

Body check: Be aware of your shoulders and relax them as you do this movement. If there is an area that feels achy or tight, breathe into that spot to let go of tension. To do that, as you inhale visualize bringing oxygen to the tight area, and as you exhale breathe out the tension. Notice if one side feels tighter than the other; what do you do differently on that side of the body? If you hear cracks or pops, it's just tension being released from the joints.

As you do the neck rolls, you may find that you want to sigh or moan or groan. Please do! This helps relieve tension and makes your jaw and facial muscles relax.

Repetitions: Two or more times on each side

Shoulder Rolls

Shoulder rolls open up the chest and upper back and relieve tension in the shoulders. It's a great movement for moms who hold their baby in a front carrier. You can do these whenever you feel the need.

Where's Baby: Next to you or in your lap

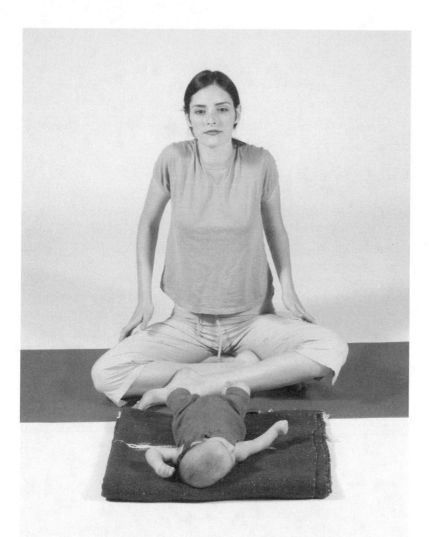

To begin: Bring your shoulders back, inhale and lift the shoulders up. Then exhale and bring the shoulders forward and down.

Body check: Enjoy an open chest when the shoulders are back, and an open back as the shoulders come forward.

Repetitions: Three circles in each direction

Forward Neck Release

This movement releases tension in your neck, shoulders and upper back. It also provides a nice stretch for the vertebrae in the cervical spine (neck).

Where's Baby: Lying beside you or in your lap

To begin: Stretch your arms out in front of you and interlace your fingers, your palms facing away from your body. Stretch your palms forward. You will feel your shoulder blades come away from each other, giving the upper back a nice stretch.

Next, raise your interlaced fingers up toward the ceiling, stretching them slightly behind your head. Then bring your palms to the

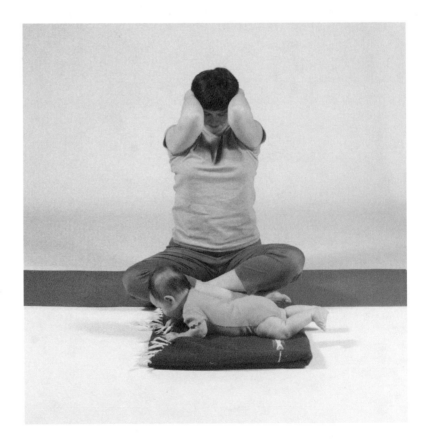

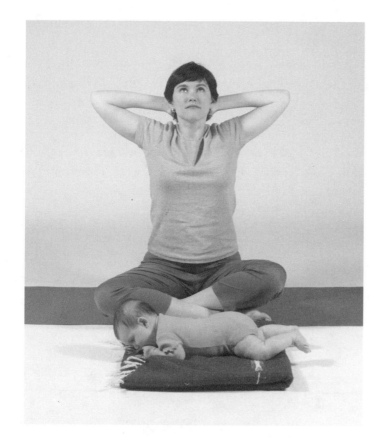

back of your head, with your elbows open to the side; feel a lovely expansion through your chest and back. Inhale. Now exhale and bring your elbows forward but not touching, so they point straight ahead. Bring your chin down toward your chest. Feel the space open up at the bottom of your neck. Hold this position for three breaths, feeling the tension release. Breathe slowly through your nose, with each exhale releasing stress and tension and each inhale creating energy and well-being. Inhale, raising the head back up. Open up the elbows and slowly look up.

Body check: Take a few breaths when your head is down and then when your head is up. Enjoy!

Repetitions: Do the entire sequence two or three times.

Foot Stretch

This stretch loosens your calf muscles, encourages blood circulation in your lower limbs and minimizes swelling in the feet and ankles. Foot stretches are very important to do if you are confined to bed after a C-section.

Where's Baby: Hold your baby or rest her in your lap. As you wiggle your toes, you can wiggle hers as well as you rotate her ankles gently and play games with her toes.

To begin: Give all your toes a nice wiggle. Feel them warm up as blood enters the tips (this is also great to do if your feet are ever cold). Rotate your ankles gently to the right, making a slow clockwise circle. Now rotate in the other direction. Do a total of five circles in each direction.

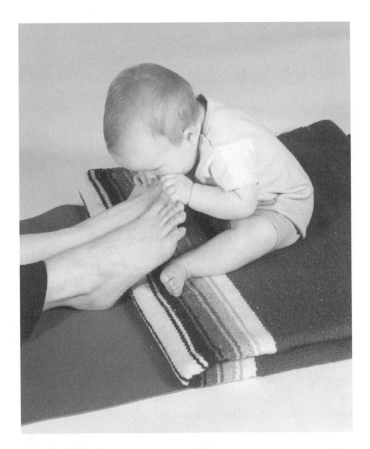

Next, flex your feet, stretching your heels away from you as you point your toes toward yourself. Hold for several seconds and release. Do this flex exercise for about one minute.

Now, stand up and stretch your toes like duck feet, imagining webs between the toes. Lift your toes off the floor and then return them to the floor, two to three times for each foot.

Body check: Make sure your whole body is comfortable as you do these movements. Remember not to point your toes, which can give you cramps (while flexing your feet can help release cramps). We tend to neglect the feet, so take some time to do these.

Don't be surprised if your feet are bigger after pregnancy. Mine went from size eight to size nine after my daughter Rachel was born, but didn't expand after Mikela's birth, thank goodness. Pregnancy also tends to flatten out feet. In standing poses you can lift your toes off the floor during a stretch—this will create an arch.

Repetitions: Stretch both feet for about one minute per foot. Do foot circles five times in each direction or as often as you desire.

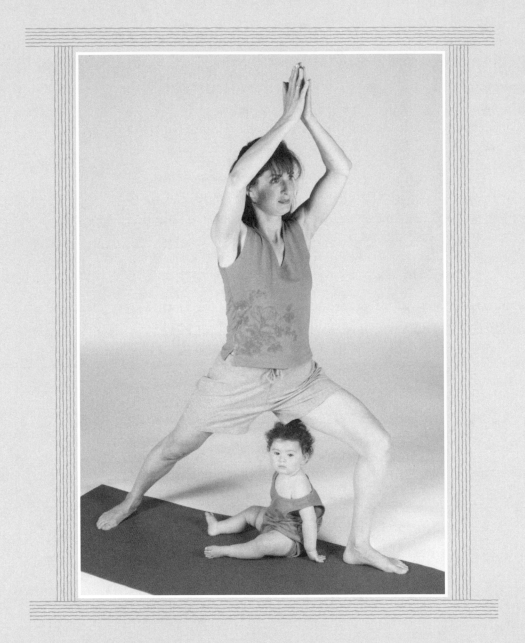

Six

Get Strong!

Strong muscles will grow fatigued more slowly and will allow you to have greater control over your movements. Strength is especially crucial during pregnancy, when your skeletal system must support not only added weight but weight distributed differently on your body. Yoga helps build and maintain important muscle sets—in the back, abdomen and pelvic area—to decrease backache, support healthy posture and contribute to your strength during labor.

After you give birth, your abdominal and pelvic floor muscles may feel stretched, unsupportive and slack, like "everything's going to fall out." That's a normal feeling. These muscles did a lot of work, so they will feel sore and maybe soft. Some new moms say about their abdominals: "What abdominals?" Yoga postures and movements will also strengthen and help tone these important muscles.

Get Strong:
To restore lost muscle tone
To regain strength and control
To improve balance
To reshape your body
To feel confident and healthy
To assert yourself physically as well as mentally

Kegels

Kegels are exercises to strengthen the pelvic floor muscles, a band of muscles between the pubic bone and the coccyx. This area has three orifices: the urethra, vagina and anus. The pelvic floor muscles surround and support these orifices and internal organs (the bladder, uterus, bowels and intestines). The pelvic floor has strength and stretch, and it is very important, especially for pregnant women and new mothers, to work these muscles to maintain the integrity of the structure.

To find your kegel muscle, imagine you are urinating and someone walks in. The muscle you use to stop the flow of urine is the kegel muscle. (However, do not practice this while urinating—this can cause urinary-tract infections.) You can feel these muscles in particular when you are in the child's pose or doing squats.

Prenatal Kegels

Having strong muscles here is important, because as the uterus gets heavier with the growing baby there is more pressure on the pelvic floor. This movement also improves pelvic blood circulation.

To begin: As you inhale slowly, lift your kegel muscle up. As you exhale slowly, release down. Then try inhaling and lifting up; keep breathing as you hold the muscle up there (three breaths) and then release. Do slowly.

Belly check: Be aware of using these muscles during lovemaking by tightening the muscle around the penis.

Repetitions: It is suggested that you do fifty to two hundred of these per day, or as many as you are comfortable doing.

Elevators

Elevators also strengthen the muscles of the pelvic floor and bring improved blood circulation to the area. It is important to work these muscles not only to build strength but also because a stronger muscle stretches more easily. In this movement you will also learn how to relax this muscle, which you do during the pushing stage of labor.

To begin: Inhale; life pelvic muscles up to first floor, second floor, third floor; exhale. Slowly lower down: third floor, second floor, first floor. The elevator floors are a visualization to squeeze the muscle a little tighter and higher. These can be done anywhere, anytime, sitting or standing.

Belly check: Keep breathing as you hold the kegel muscle up.

Repetitions: Two

Kegels After Birth

These are important to perform right after delivery (and for the rest of your life). While you may not feel like doing them immediately after delivery because your pelvic floor is sore and swollen, trust me—kegels will make you feel better. If you've had an episiotomy or had a tear during childbirth, kegels will bring extra circulation to the area, helping you to heal. One of my students waited three weeks after she gave birth to begin her kegel exercises. She then regretted waiting so long—by that time, she told me, everything already felt like it was going to fall out. Please start doing these as soon as possible!

Where's Baby: In your arms, at your side or with a partner, family member or caregiver

To begin: From a seated or lying position inhale slowly and lift the kegel muscle up. Exhale and slowly bring it down. Inhale, lift the muscle up and hold for a few seconds while still breathing. Exhale and bring the muscle down.

Body check: Don't hold your breath while doing kegels. You can also try exhaling as you lift up the pelvic floor muscles and inhaling as you release them.

Repetitions: Believe it or not, it is recommended to do two hundred a day. Do them—they are important!

The prenatal exercises connected through to postpartum. And postpartum has been phenomenal for my body for a speedier recovery. The strengthening helps in terms of abdominal awareness. You get so exhausted, it helps with lifting the baby well, getting up from the floor with the baby, moving and carrying the baby—especially as he gets heavier—so it doesn't hurt me.

—ELIZABETH AND SON ALEXANDER

Get Strong!

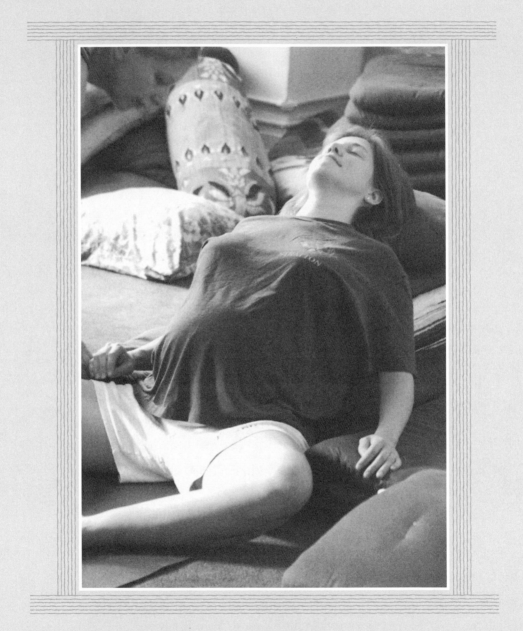

Seven

Before Your Baby Arrives: Prenatal Yoga

Prenatal yoga adapts some traditional yoga postures—asanas—in order to meet the needs and changes of pregnancy. The asanas gently build strength and flexibility. There are no high-impact movements to strain or overwhelm you. The poses help you maintain fitness as your body grows with a new life, and through specific exercises prepare you for labor and delivery and afterward. The asanas also offer ways to release tension without strain and to find calm in a time of physical and emotional change.

You can do the asanas as a series or you can mix and match, depending on how you feel on a particular day and your time constraints. Perform all the movements gently, never forcing a stretch. Listen to your body to best determine how long to hold a stretch, the number of repetitions and which asanas to do on a particular day. During the movements, breathe in slowly through your nose*, feeling the breath coming in, and then breathe out gently through

*Traditionally in yoga, all breath is in through the nose and out through the nose. During pregnancy, if you prefer to exhale through an open mouth, go for it—you will be exhaling through the mouth during labor. Also allow yourself to make sounds with the exhalations, as this can release additional tension.

your nose. Connect one breath to another, fluidly and rhythmically. During the exercises, focus on breathing and relaxation—above all, don't forget to breathe!

Prenatal Routines

During a prenatal class I will lead my students through different poses on different days. However, I follow a standard flow: we begin with breathing and warm-up, do some floor postures (such as wag the tail, cat and cow and pelvic rolls), do a twist, perform our kegels, do squats, standing and balancing poses, and finish up with relaxation poses. On some days you may feel like doing a long routine, on others perhaps just some breathing or a few warm-ups. Or you might want to go right to relaxation! Listen to your body to decide what you want to do, and as you find your favorite poses, mix and match to create your own routines.

As you go through your pregnancy you will experience physical changes each day that will affect which postures are comfortable to do. Some women, for example, love downward dog throughout their pregnancy; others stop at seven months because the position becomes uncomfortable. Do what feels right. Always be aware of your posture and breath and learn to work with your abdominal and pelvic floor muscles.

For my avid yogi mamas, challenge yourself. Do moon salutations (page 224) and do plank (page 80) but also let yourself melt into supported bound angle (supta baadha konasana).

Begin in a seated position (cross-legged if it is comfortable for you).

Half Neck Rolls

Half neck rolls relieve tension in the neck and shoulders. I do these many times a day. Please do at least three on each side.

Stay seated (or stand if that is more comfortable) and move into shoulder rolls.

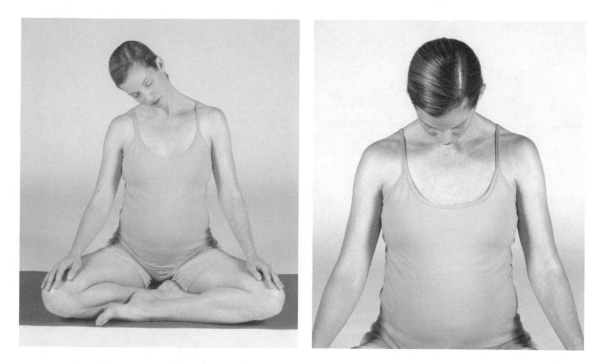

*I have put down approximate lengths for the routines; however, please don't get attached to the length of time. For some of you it may be shorter, for others longer, depending on how long your body asks you to stay in each posture.

Before Your
Baby Arrives:
Prenatal Yoga

Shoulder Rolls

Shoulder rolls open up the chest and upper back and relieve tension in the shoulders. This movement also helps relieve the "turtle back" posture that many people have. Make three circles in each direction.

Come onto your hands and knees.

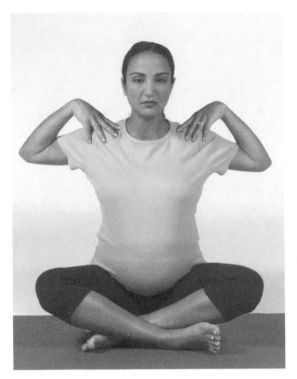

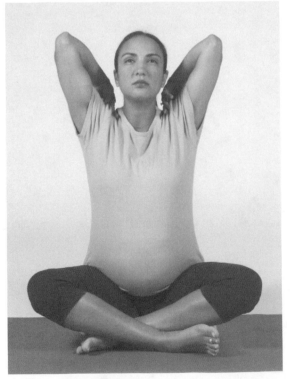

Wag the Tail

This movement gives a good stretch to the muscles between the ribs.

To begin: Come onto your hands and knees. Position your palms under your shoulders and your knees under your hips. Use your abdominals to hug your baby. Inhale. As you exhale, look over your right shoulder as you push out your right hip, bringing your right shoulder and right hip toward each other. Inhale back to center. Exhale and repeat on the left side.

Belly check: Hug your baby with your abdominal muscles as you do this posture and contract the pelvic floor.

Repetitions: Three times on each side

Stay on your hands and knees and move into cat and cow.

I started yoga prenatally because I felt tension in my neck. It's made me more flexible—I noticed when I was pregnant I was always more comfortable on yoga days.

—JODY AND DAUGHTER SIMONE

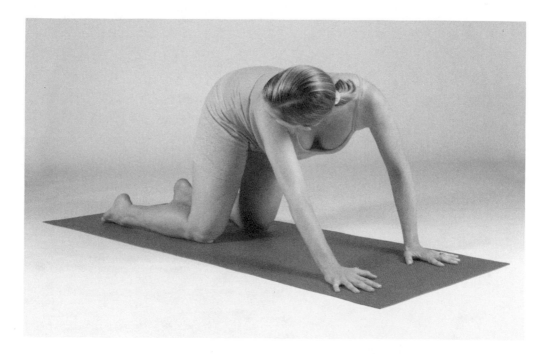

Cat and Cow

Cat and cow pose keeps the spine flexible and strengthens your abdominal muscles. This relaxing and energizing movement is great for relieving lower-back aches.

To begin: Stay on your hands and knees. This is a great position, because the weight of the uterus and baby is no longer pressing against your lower back. Do not lock your elbows. Inhale. As you exhale, move your pelvis slightly back and down.

Now let your head hang down so you are looking at your knees. Use your abdominals here; hug your baby by bringing your belly button up toward your baby. Inhale, bringing your pelvis slightly forward as you lengthen your spine and lift your head gently, looking up. Exhale and repeat.

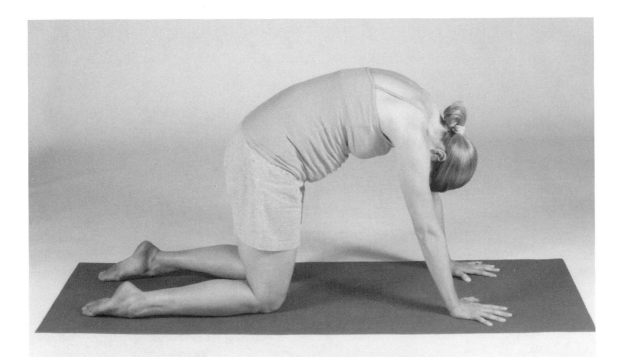

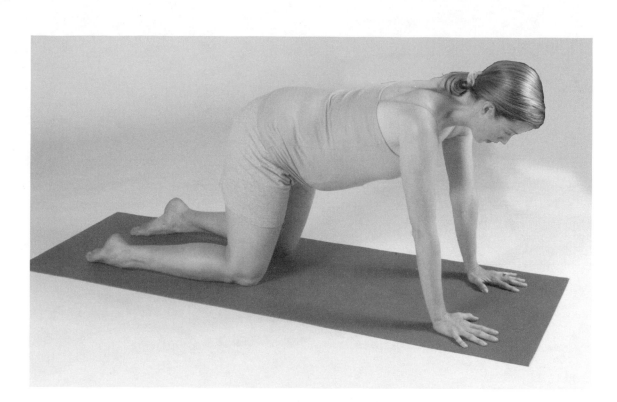

Belly check: Be aware of the motion coming from the pelvis; you are lengthening the spine by moving your buttocks and pelvis backward and down, and forward and up, not arching your back.

Repetitions: Three times

Stay on all fours.

Pigeon

Pigeon pose is an excellent hip opener and is good for sciatica.

To begin: Start on all fours. Bring your right knee forward, and move your right calf and ankle in front of your left knee, as you extend your left leg straight back, top of foot to floor. Prop yourself up with your arms, then slowly lower forward onto your forearms and then bring your forehead to the floor. You can always put a

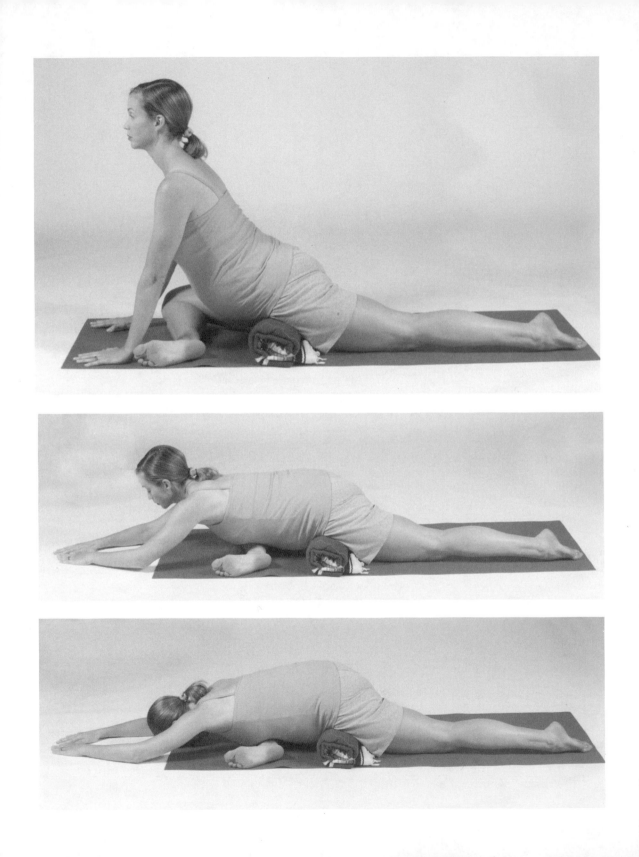

blanket under your pelvis or buttock to ease the stretch. Hold for three breaths. Slowly come back up and back to all fours. Repeat on the other side.

Belly check: As your belly gets bigger, just do the leg position if it is uncomfortable to bring your arms and forehead to the floor.

Repetitions: Once on each side, holding for three breaths

Come back onto all fours, bring your right leg forward, bring your hand to your thigh and come into a standing position.

Squats

Squats strengthen the legs and open up the pelvic area, improving circulation in the region. This asana allows the lower back to lengthen. It is also a good way to get from the floor to a standing position.

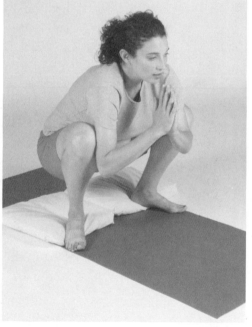

In the last few weeks of pregnancy this asana helps the baby's head to engage, the point at which the baby descends into the pelvic cavity. Some women deliver in this position, as it works with gravity to birth a baby.

Medical cautions: Do not do squats if you have varicose veins, hemorrhoids or placenta previa. If your baby is in breech position, do not do after your thirty-sixth week (you can do the child's pose instead).

To begin: Inhale. As you exhale, bend your knees and bring them over your toes. Lower your buttocks toward the floor. Make sure the soles of your feet are flat on the floor as you go into your squat. (If you need support in a squat, you can use the wall as support for your back. If your heels do not come to the floor, place a blanket or cushion under your heels.) Bring your hands into a prayer position, with your elbows inside your knees. Keep your back straight. If this position is too strenuous on your legs, sit on a pillow. Hold for one minute. Then bring your hands behind you, sit on your buttocks and stretch your legs out, moving them up and down to release any tension, or you can come from your squat to standing.

Belly check: Be aware of the lovely stretch in your lower back.

Repetitions: Once, increasing how long you hold the squat as you get more comfortable in this position. This is a great position to do many times a day, particularly if you've been standing or sitting too long. It helps with lower-back ache.

Come onto your hands and knees.

Child's Pose

The child's pose is a terrific position for just relaxing, letting your body and mind settle into serenity. The stretch opens up the pelvic area, gently stretches the lower back, and expands the chest and back.

To begin: From your hands and knees, open your knees a little wider, bringing your toes together and your heels apart. Move your buttocks back to rest between your heels, bringing your forehead down toward the floor. As your belly gets bigger, you can put a pillow under your forehead. Breathe and relax. You can keep your arms crossed under your forehead, stretched straight above your head or stretched out along your body—whichever you find most comfortable.

Rest in this position for as long as you like. Feel the gentle stretch in the lower back. Concentrate on slow, rhythmic breathing.

When you are ready, walk your hands up to the chest and inhale into a sitting position. Or from your hands and knees, come onto your knees, bring one foot to the floor, curl back the toes of your back leg and come up to standing.

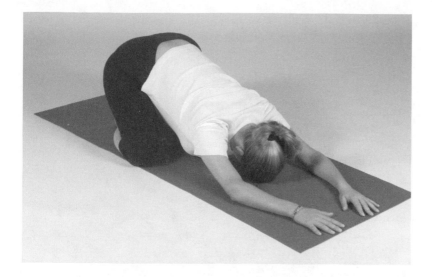

Belly check: Here are some variations to make this pose as comfortable as possible:

- If your belly feels squished, try opening your knees wider.
- Place a blanket between your buttocks and calves.
- Put a blanket under your knees (an essential if done on a bare floor) to cushion your knees and ankles.
- You can also put a blanket under your chest (right above your breasts) to give your belly more room.
- If you don't feel comfortable coming down all the way, come onto your forearms.

Repetitions: Once or as many times as you like throughout the day

Staying in child's pose, begin kegels. Then it's time to relax.

Supported Bound Angle (Supta Baddha Konasana)

This is a terrific position for quick rejuvenation. The pose opens up the chest as well as the hip and groin area, encouraging blood flow. It also helps alleviate backaches. Hold as long as you want.

Medical cautions: Do not do this pose if you have any nerve problems in your neck or spinal disk conditions.

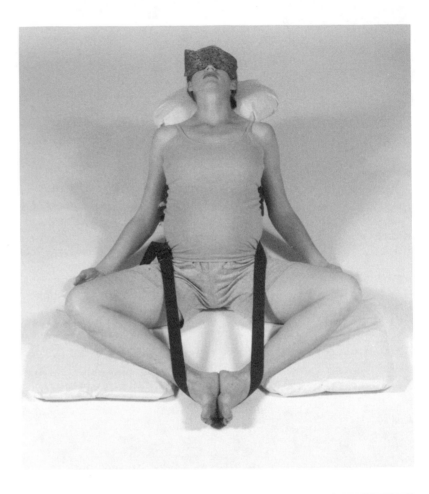

Start in a seated position.

Shoulder Rolls

Do three shoulder rolls forward and three shoulder rolls back.

Side Bends

Side bends are great for stretching your side muscles from the neck down to the pelvis, for opening up the chest and upper back, for realigning the spine and for toning the waist.

To begin: Sit comfortably, checking your posture to make sure both buttocks are touching the floor. Interlace your fingers, palms away from you, and stretch your arms out in front. Inhale, lift your arms toward the ceiling, expanding your rib cage, chest and upper back. Exhale, and place your hands behind your head. Bring your elbows out to the sides, stretching your shoulders and opening up your chest. Inhale. On the exhale, bend to the right. Bring your right hand down, palm to the floor, and walk your fingers out. Hold the stretch for three breaths, then inhale and come back to center. When you are sitting up straight again, exhale and repeat on the left side.

Body check: Do not arch your lower back. Keep your sits bones grounded to the floor.

Repetitions: Two to three times to each side

Stand up for pelvic rolls.

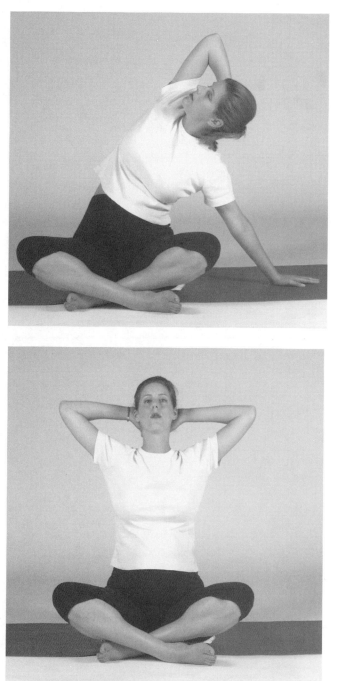

Pelvic Rolls

Pelvic rolls relieve lower-back achiness and strengthen the abdominal muscles.

To begin: Stand with your feet a little more than hip width apart. Bend your knees slightly. Push your hips and pelvis out toward the right. Then bring your pelvis back. Next move your hips to the left and bring your pubic bone forward. This is one complete circle. Do two more continuous clockwise cycles, then switch directions.

Belly check: Be aware of your posture; make sure your knees are bent slightly. You can massage your belly as you do these.

Repetitions: Three circles on each side

Come down onto your hands and knees for child's pose.

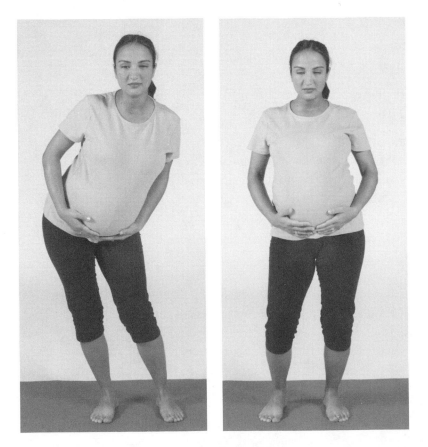

Child's Pose

Relax in child's pose, then begin kegels.

Bring your chin into your chest and roll up to a sitting position.

Diamond Pose

The diamond pose gives the upper leg muscles a nice stretch. It's also a good pose for indigestion.

To begin: From child's pose, bring your chin into your chest, walk your hands in and come up to a seated position or diamond pose. Relax your breathing. Hold for five breaths. You may want to put a blanket under your legs and ankles or between your buttocks and calves.

Belly check: Do not do this if it feels uncomfortable.

Repetitions: Do once.

Bring your legs out from underneath you and stretch them out. Then stand up.

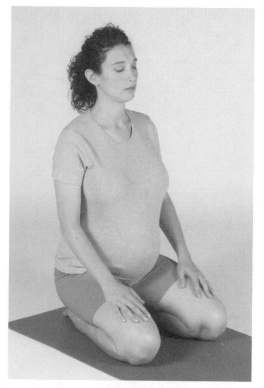

Pelvic Tilts

Pelvic tilts strengthen muscles in your lower back, buttocks and abdomen and tone muscles to contribute to healthy circulation.

To begin: Stand against a wall. Bend your knees, pushing your back against the wall; your feet will move about two feet away. As you inhale, lift your pelvis away from the wall. As you bring your pelvis forward, squeeze your buttocks together. Exhale slowly and bring the pelvis back to the wall by rolling down the vertebrae and bringing your belly button back toward your baby and the wall.

Belly check: Feel a gentle massage in your lower back as you bring your pelvis back to the wall.

Repetitions: Begin with six and and raise the number of repetitions as you like.

Legs Up Wall

This gentle inversion lets blood and fluids flow from the lower body in the opposite direction. It's good for tired, swollen legs or ankles and helps varicose veins. My pregnant moms usually love doing this pose, but some find it uncomfortable toward the end of pregnancy.

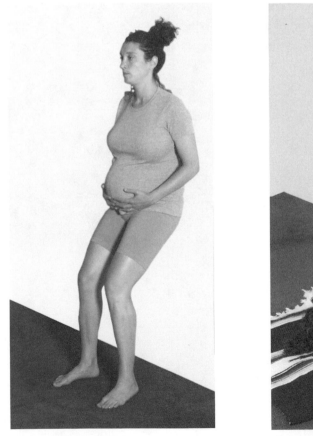
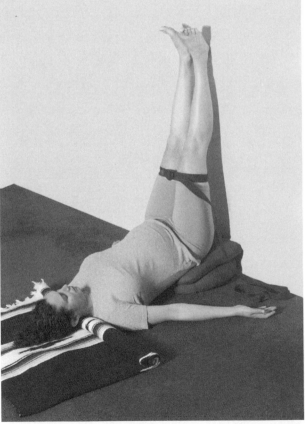

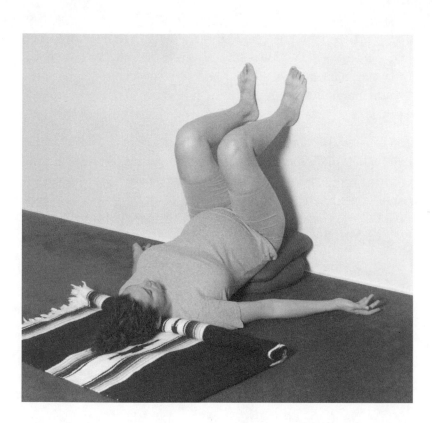

To begin: Sit on a cushion an inch away from the wall. Swing around and bring your legs up the wall as you lie back, with your hips on the cushion. Make sure your hips are on the cushion so your pelvis is off the floor and higher than your head. Breathe deeply in this position for five minutes. If you feel dizzy, walk your legs down the wall and relax on your left side.

Belly check: When I was pregnant and big, I didn't like this pose. I felt "suffocated" by my breasts and belly. Of course, if you find this pose uncomfortable, please don't do it.

Repetitions: Hold for up to five minutes.

Butterfly Pose

The butterfly pose opens up the pelvis and hip joints. It also increases circulation to the entire genital area.

To begin: Bend your knees and bring the soles of your feet together. Let your knees come down toward the floor, but do not bounce. (You may want pillows under your knees for additional support.) Breathe normally, relaxing into the pose. Feel a connection to the earth.

You can also try coming into a forward bend from this position. Inhale, exhale and hinge forward from the hips, leading out with the crown of your head and lengthening through the spine. Bring your hands down to the floor, relaxing the head, neck and shoulders. Breathe, relax and when you're ready, come out of the forward bend by inhaling and coming up, lengthening through the crown

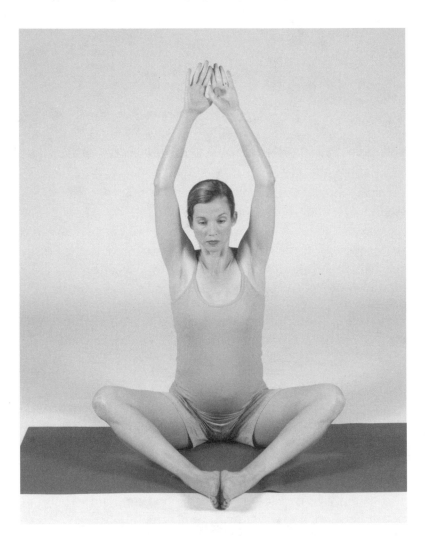

Yoga Mom,
Buddha Baby

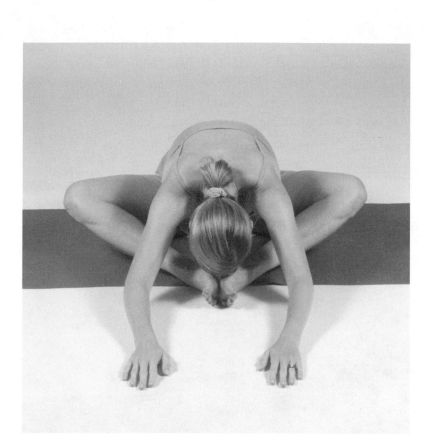

of the head. This forward bend can also be done with your legs open in the V position.

Belly check: Keep the asana comfortable. As your belly gets bigger you may not want to come down as far.

Repetitions: Once, holding for eight to ten breaths

Stretch out legs and then come into a cross-legged position.

Spinal Twist

Eastern medical practitioners believe that by twisting the spine, you squeeze out toxins from the spine and help refresh the kidneys, spleen and adrenal glands. Spinal twists also keep the spine flexible while working the abdominal muscles, and they release upper- and middle-back aches. This is a very gentle twist.

To begin: Sit in a cross-legged position. To check your posture, draw your sits bones to the floor while keeping your spine lengthened. Inhale and bring your left palm to your right knee, bringing your right hand behind you. Exhale and start twisting to the right. As you do, look over your right shoulder. Feel the flexibility of the spine. Breathe, and as you exhale see if your breath moves you a little farther into the twist. Inhale and slowly come back to center. Exhale and repeat on the left side.

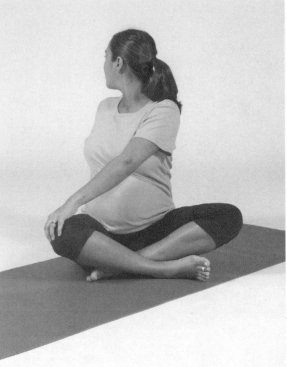

Belly check: Be aware of keeping both buttocks on the floor. Allow the shoulders and jaw to relax.

Repetitions: Once each side, holding for three breaths

Lie down.

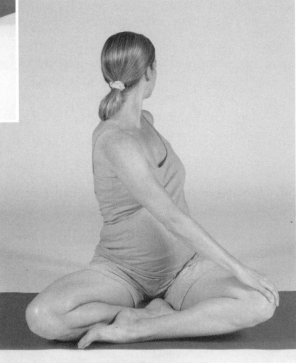

Reclining Buddha

This comfortable, relaxing position is just about letting go. Stay here as long as you like.

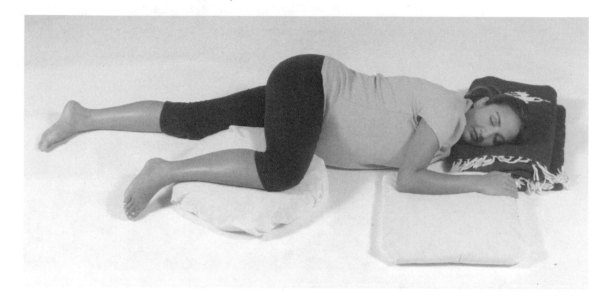

Begin in a seated position (cross-legged if it is comfortable for you).

Three-Part Breath (Deergha Swaasam)

This breathing brings calmness into the body. It also increases energy and vitality by bringing more oxygen into the lungs. Deergha Swaasam also helps turn your awareness to the abdominal muscles as you concentrate on breathing in and out. This type of breathing can be practiced whenever you feel a need to center yourself. Do for at least six breaths.

If you are lying down, sit up.

Before Your Baby Arrives: Prenatal Yoga

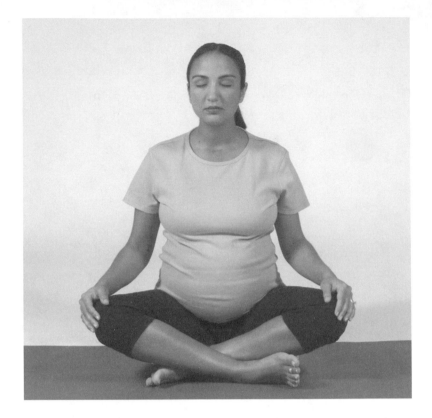

Half Neck Roll

Do three half neck rolls.

Shoulder Roll

Do three shoulder rolls.

Spinal Twist

Do a twist to each side.

Come onto your hands and knees.

Wag the Tail

Do three on each side.

Cat and Cow

Do three flows of this movement.

Child's Pose

Relax in child's pose, then begin kegels.

Sit up and then come onto your hands and knees.

Downward Dog

This is a terrific stretching movement for the back and hamstrings. Downward dog also strengthens the upper body and tones your abdominals.

To begin: Begin on your hands and knees. Make sure to open up between your fingers. Inhale, exhale and push up, moving your buttocks toward the ceiling in an inverted V. Bring your belly button toward your baby and bring your heels down toward the floor. Open up between your shoulder blades, let your head relax and look at your knees.

Time: Stay in this position for three breaths.

Variation: While in downward dog, bend your left knee. Now bring the right heel down toward the floor and hold for ten seconds. Then bend your right knee and bring your left heel to the floor, holding for ten seconds. Finish by bringing both heels back down toward the floor.

When you are ready to come out of the downward dog, you can either come back to your hands and knees or come into plank.

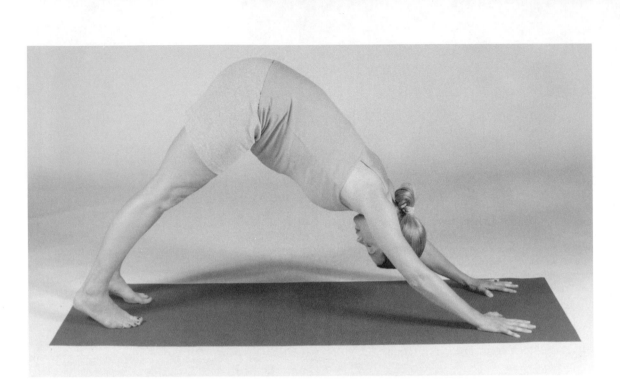

Belly check: Be aware of the feet and legs, bringing them close together. Let the shoulders relax. Make sure not to lock your elbows (hyperextension weakens the ligaments).

Repetitions: Do once.

Plank Pose

This advanced pose strengthens your arms, back and abdominal muscles. If you are a beginner, please don't do this pose.

To begin: Come into plank from downward dog. Lower your hips, so you are as straight as a plank. Your hands are directly under your shoulders. Tighten your abdominal and buttocks muscles, pressing back through your heels. Gaze at the floor. Hold for three breaths.

Belly check: Don't let your hips sink or your buttocks rise up. Make sure not to lock your elbows.

Yoga Mom,
Buddha Baby

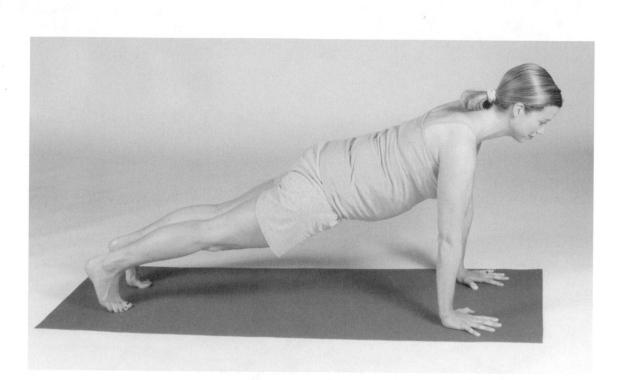

Repetitions: Hold for three breaths.

From plank, come onto all fours and up to standing. From standing, move into triangle pose.

Triangle

The triangle pose strengthens and tones legs and buttock muscles while giving a nice overall stretch. To prevent sliding, it's good to do it on a yoga mat. You can also do this pose against a wall for extra support.

To begin: From a standing position, step your feet one leg length apart; be comfortable, so you feel grounded. Face your left foot forward, the right to the right side, with your hips facing forward. Stretch your arms out to each side, parallel to the floor, feeling your back and chest open up. Inhale, exhale and reach out to the right side. Inhale, raising the left arm up. Exhale slowly, bringing your right arm down against the right leg. Keep your left hip back

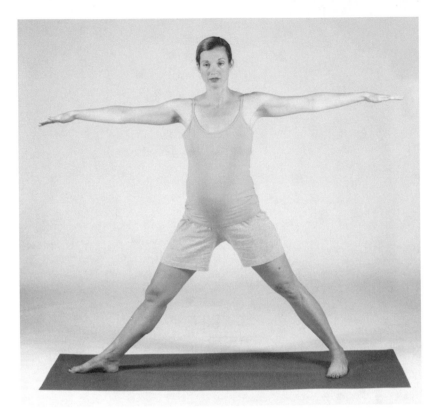

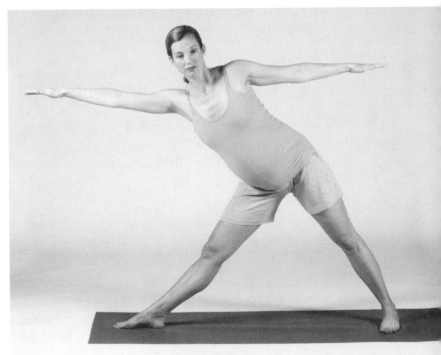

Yoga Mom,
Buddha Baby

or open (this is where the wall helps). You can look up toward the raised palm. Breathe.

It does not matter how far you come over, but it is important to maintain the feeling of being grounded. To do this, press down through the legs and make sure your shoulders and arms are relaxed. Keep the left hip and chest open.

Come out of triangle when you are ready, grounding your feet and inhaling up to center. Move your right foot forward and left foot to the side, and repeat to the left.

Variation: You can bend your knee during the stretch if you get tired, with your knee fully extended.

Belly check: It doesn't matter how far over on the right leg you go; just make sure you get a side stretch. Keep the left hip back, again working the side stretch. Check your posture when you get back to a standing position.

Repetitions: Once on both sides, holding for three breaths

Walk to a wall.

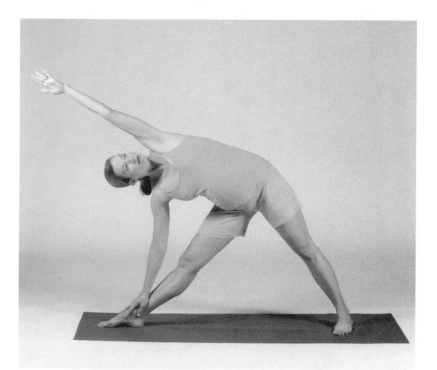

Right Angle Stretch

This is a great stretch for the legs, back and arms, plus it lengthens the spine. You can also do this with a partner; you can get a deeper stretch as your partner gently brings your pelvis toward him.

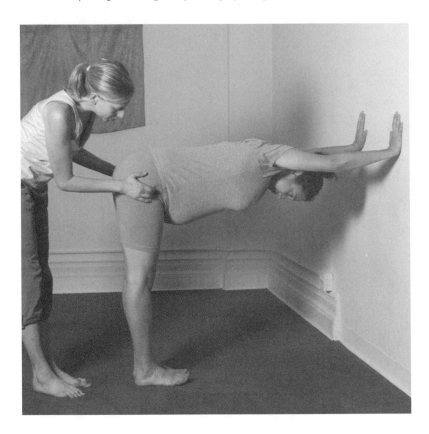

To begin: Stand an arm's length away from a wall. Walk your arms down the wall with your feet away from the wall until your arms are parallel to the floor and your legs parallel to the wall. Bring your back perpendicular to the wall. Readjust your feet if necessary to bring them close together—a few inches—but not touching. Gaze down toward the floor. Inhale and exhale, feeling as though your buttocks are being pulled toward the wall behind you as you are pushing the wall in front of you away from yourself. You can bend your left knee as you push your right heel into the floor. Then switch sides.

Belly check: Make sure that your legs are parallel and your back perpendicular to the wall so that you make a right angle with your body.

Variation: This stretch also works well if you lean into a kitchen counter, so try it while making dinner.

Repetitions: As many times during the day as needed. Hold for three breaths.

Come away from the wall and stand.

Squats

Hold the squat for ten breaths.

Medical caution: If after week thirty-six your baby is in breech position, do not do squats. Do not do squats if you have varicose veins, hemorrhoids or placenta previa.

Bring your hands behind you, come onto your buttocks in a seated position and stretch out your legs.

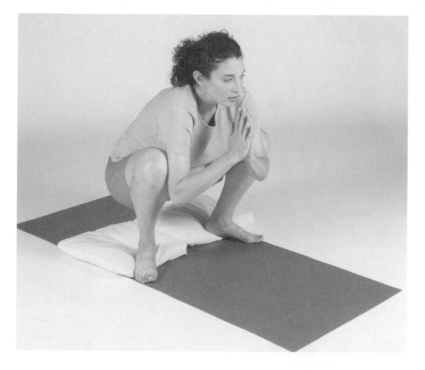

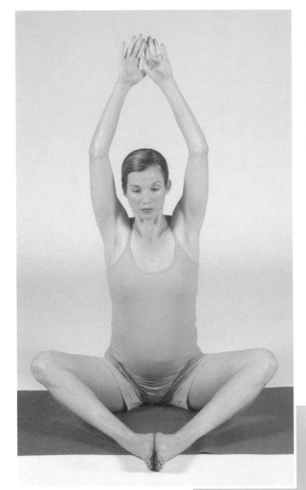

Butterfly Pose

Hold for five breaths.

Stretch out your legs in front of you, bring them around to one side and come onto your hands and knees.

Child's Pose

Time for more kegels!

End your routine in a relaxation pose.

Side Lying Position

Hold as long as you like.

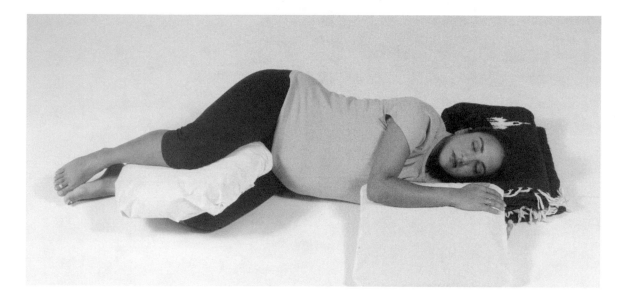

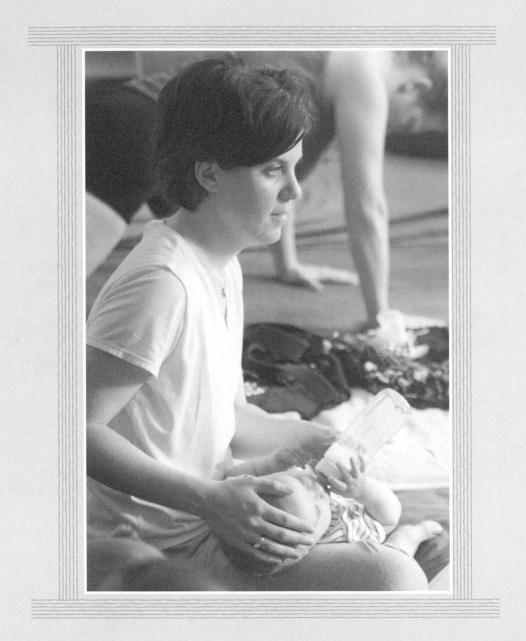

Eight

After Your
Baby Is Born

No one can tell you what to expect once your baby is born; until you've done it, you don't quite know what the experience will be like. It's blissful, amazing, overwhelming and emotional, all at the same time. When there's a new baby, the energy is so special, it's something close to mystical. I like to think there's a universal mother (an energy) that looks after us all.

For some reason I thought the days after giving birth would be easier than they were, which is crazy, because real transformation is never easy. The births of my children were the two most amazing days of my life. All women have amazing birth stories.

Motherhood is both a very individual experience and a very universal one; you can make yoga a part of it in a way that is comfortable for you. Some women start a few very simple breathing exercises and postures as soon as one day after giving birth; I always tell my moms to start kegels right away. Others wait up to six weeks after their postdelivery checkup before beginning yoga. If you do not feel ready, or if some postures do not feel right immediately, then try again in a few days or a week. But don't leave it for too long! Remember, the kegels are really important to do now, to strengthen the pelvic floor. If you've had an episiotomy or ripped,

Postpartum Blues

Yoga can help with feelings of depression and of being overwhelmed and anxious—babies are very demanding, and you may have a feeling of losing yourself. Because hormones are raging after one gives birth, all of these feelings may be present. Even ten minutes a day of mindful breathing will help. Of course, if you can, give yourself longer (an hour is ideal, though any time investment is of great benefit).

Please ask for help if you need it. Our culture is not one that supports mothers and babies as others do, but mothers and babies are sacred. They need to be fed and taken care of. There is a great energy around moms and babies. For a partner, it is a time to give unconditional love and support. In India, family and friends look after moms for twenty-two days following their giving birth. In some European countries maternity leave is for a full year and fathers get paternity leave. New mothers deserve extra attention.

you'll heal quicker, as kegels bring more blood to this area. You can also use the many hours you spend feeding your baby to breathe fully and consciously, allowing yourself to be calm and to relax.

Birth to Six Weeks

After being in a state of pregnancy for nine months, your body is now beginning to change back to the way it was before. Hormonal changes abound, and depending on your labor, it may take time to get your strength back. While doing yoga, pay particular attention to working the abdominal muscles, because they have been stretched out by the uterus. You will also want to start kegels to get your pelvic floor muscles toned. It is important to get stronger, because your baby's weight is only going to increase. And during this time your baby is getting used to being here. She will be in your arms a lot; it is a time of bonding. As you do your yoga, talk to her—babies love to hear the sound of their mother's voice.

All of the following positions and exercises are safe for women who have recently given birth. A woman who has had a vaginal birth might start right away. While the postures are safe for a woman who has had a cesarean, she may want to wait a little longer. To decide when to start, listen to your body.

Any asana can be performed alone or in conjunction with any other movement. I have provided some series of movements that incorporate stretches, strengthening and breathing to give a fluid all-body routine. The series begin with gentle warm-ups and end with relaxation poses.

Be aware of:

- After giving birth, use your abdominal and pelvic floor muscles when you walk around.
- It is very important to work your kegels now.
- Kabaalabhahti breathing helps get anesthesia out of your system.
- The postures are safe for C-section births—again, listen to your body to know when to do something and when not to.
- Take time in between each pose to breathe and to listen to your body.

I believe that women who have practiced yoga during pregnancy come into postpartum with a stronger body, but even more important, a good understanding of their body. Many moms ask me, "Will I ever wear my jeans again?" Yes, but not right after giving birth. Remember, it took you nine months to get to this place. Please don't be horrified by your pouch, sometimes referred to affectionately as "jelly belly," or your abdominals, sometimes called "God's girdle." By gently working the abdominals after giving birth, your jelly belly won't last long. I'd like to share that since giving birth to my daughters, I am twenty pounds heavier than before, but I think I need it. Now I'm curvaceous. So please learn to love that belly and your abdominals, and be good to yourself during this time.

I was having some postpartum anxieties. The yoga exercise made me feel like I was getting my strength back, and the relaxations were awesome. Stretching helped me reconnect with my body. It was amazing how the labor had zapped my energy.

—VIRGINIA AND
DAUGHTER MAYA

*After Your Baby
Is Born*

This important series gets you to use your pelvic floor and abdominal muscles and encourages focused breathing. In the days right after giving birth, try to work up to doing the entire routine. If you do this series for the first three weeks you are doing great!

Sit comfortably or lie down. Remember to do all the movements very gently.

Three-Part Breath (Deergha Swaasam)

If your baby is agitated, pick him up and begin Deergha Swaasam, breathing with your baby. As you time your breathing to your baby's, or bring calm to your breathing, he may also begin to relax.

This breathing practice calms the body and brings energy and vitality by bringing extra oxygen into the lungs. Deergha Swaasam also helps turn your awareness to the abdominal muscles as you concentrate on breathing in and out.

This type of breathing can be practiced whenever you feel a need to center yourself. When I feel anxious or overwhelmed, I remember to breathe this way and I immediately feel better. It is particularly nice to practice this breathing while feeding or holding your baby. The baby picks up on the calmness and positive feeling.

Where's Baby: Held against your chest or in your lap

Labor just took everything out of me—I had no strength. The yoga helped me get everything back. I quietly became stronger. The stretching and muscle-building improves strength to carry the diaper bag, stroller and baby. And Maya loves it. When she was small we did sit-ups, and she loves my hair in her face when I am doing an exercise. She's now a "Buddha Baby," very calm and peaceful. She responds to the chanting—it calms her—so we do it before bedtime, like a prayer. We have incorporated the give-and-take of doing yoga together into our relationship in all areas of our lives.

—VIRGINIA AND
DAUGHTER MAYA

*Yoga Mom,
Buddha Baby*

---

*I have put down approximate lengths for the routines; however, please don't get attached to the length of time. For some of you it may be shorter, for others longer, depending on how long your body asks you to stay in each posture.

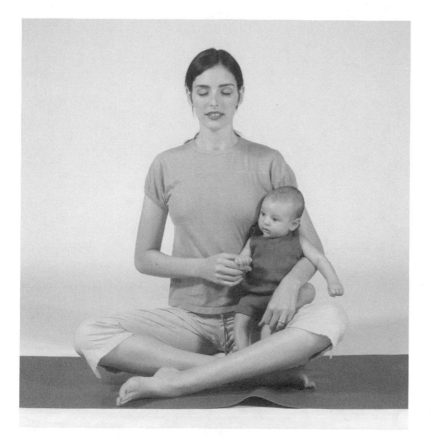

Kegels

This is worth repeating: kegels exercise your pelvic floor and are important to perform right after delivery (and for the rest of your life). You may not feel like doing these immediately after delivery because the pelvic floor is sore and swollen, but kegels will make you feel better. And if you've had an episiotomy or had a tear during childbirth, kegels will bring extra circulation to the area, helping you to heal.

Believe it or not, it is recommended to do two hundred kegels a day. So please do these important exercises!

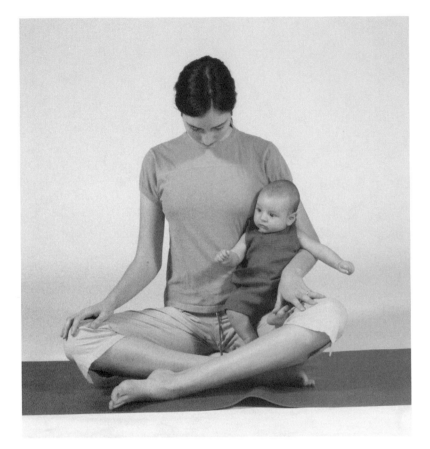

Bigger breasts, breast-feeding, bottle-feeding and carrying a baby can add tension to the back and neck muscles. Half neck rolls relieve tension in the neck and shoulders.

Be aware of your shoulders and relax them during this movement. If an area feels achy or tight, breathe into that spot to let go of tension. To do that, as you inhale visualize bringing oxygen to the tight area, and as you exhale breathe out the tension. Notice if one side feels tighter than the other; what do you do differently on that side of the body? If you hear cracks or pops, it's just tension being released from the joints.

As you do the neck rolls, you may find that you want to sigh or moan or groan. Please do! This helps relieve tension and makes your jaw and facial muscles relax.

Where's Baby: Your baby can either be in your arms or lying next to you or in your lap.

Repetitions: Two or more times on each side

Lie down on your back with your knees bent.

Pelvic Tilts

Pelvic tilts strengthen muscles in your lower back, buttocks and abdomen and tone muscles to contribute to healthy circulation.

Where's Baby: Lying on a blanket next to you

To begin: Lie down and bend your knees, keeping the soles of your feet on the floor. As you inhale, tilt your pelvis upward. Exhale

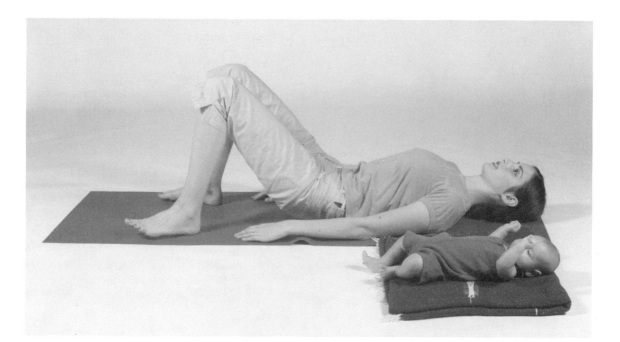

slowly and bring the pelvis back down and gently contract the abdominal muscles.

Body check: You will feel a gentle massage in your lower back as you bring your pelvis down to the floor.

C-Sections: Pelvic tilts are excellent if you have had a C-section; they can be started right away. As you exhale, contract the abdominal muscles. You may even want to bring your hand below the navel to feel the abdominal muscles as they work.

Repetitions: Begin with three and raise the number of repetitions as you feel more comfortable.

Variation with Baby (beginning at 3 to 4 weeks): Rest your baby on your belly and against your thighs. Support her with one or both hands. Babies get a fun little ride as you bring your pelvis up and down!

Stay lying down and move into abdominal work.

Abdominal Work I

You can begin these abdominal exercises for toning and strengthening right after birth. They can be done on the floor or in bed.

Where's Baby: Lying next to you

To begin: Lie down on your back. Bend your knees, keeping the soles of your feet on the floor. Cross your arms over your midsection and exhale. Contract your abdominals by bringing the belly button back to the spine and raise your head and neck off the floor. Lower yourself back down again.

Body check: While doing this movement, it is important to focus on the abs; visualize them working. Do not use your neck or other muscles to raise or lower yourself.

C-sections: Please do this with a pillow under your head.

Repetitions: Begin with five and work up to fifteen to twenty or whatever is comfortable per day.

My abdominal muscles were very strong. I imagined that after giving birth I would not be able to wear a bikini, that I would have to go into hiding, but it was amazing how fast I felt good about my body, and would show it. After two weeks I went to a swimming pool in my bikini. The exercises helped.

—TAMAR AND SON NATHANAEL

Yoga Mom,
Buddha Baby

Staying on your back, move into the bridge.

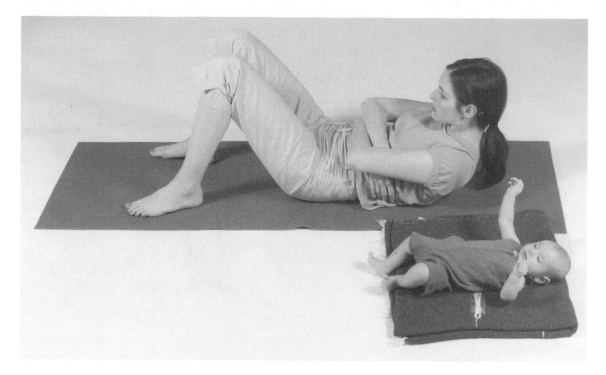

The Bridge

The bridge works the buttocks (gluteus muscle), which helps alleviate stress on the lower back. This pose also stretches the fronts of the thighs.

Where's Baby: On a blanket in front of you. (When your baby is three months old you can do this with her on your thighs.)

To begin: Lie on your back and bend your knees, keeping the soles of your feet on the floor. Bring your belly button back toward your spine, squeeze your buttocks and raise your hips off the floor (or bed). In addition to the buttocks, also lift up and contract your pelvic floor muscles. Hold this bridge pose for as long as it feels good. To come out of the posture, lower down vertebra by vertebra, bringing your pelvis to the floor.

Body check: Use your abdominals and glutes.

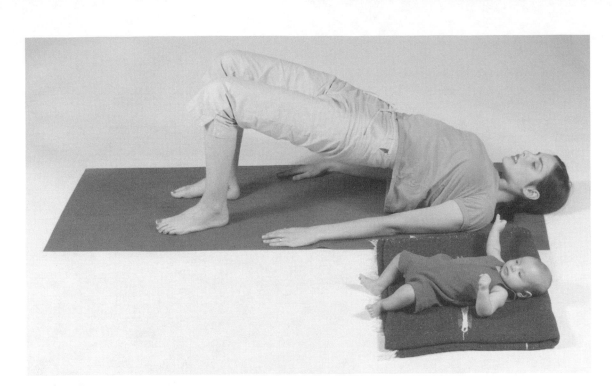

Repetitions: Do once.

Stay lying down to move into baby crocodile spinal twist.

Baby Crocodile Spinal Twist

This posture opens the chest and hips and gently stretches your spine. It's a favorite of my moms!

Where's Baby: On a blanket beside you

To begin: Lie on your back with your knees bent to your chest. Extend your arms out to the side, keeping them on the floor perpendicular to your body. Bring both knees together over to the right side of your body and turn your head to your left side. Hold this posture as long as you like. Then bring the left knee over to the other side. When the right knee doesn't stay down anymore, bring it over to the left side too. Turn your head to the right. Hold as long as you like. Bring your head and knees back to center, hold,

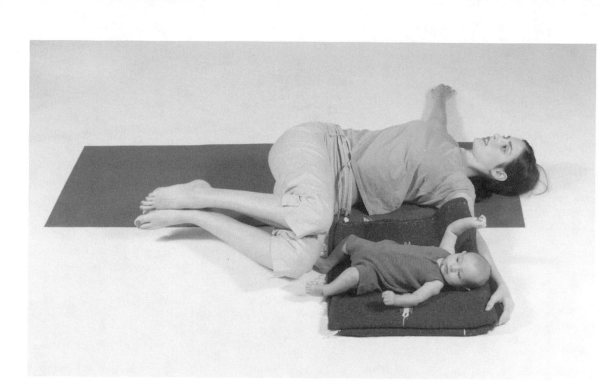

then stretch each leg all the way out, one at a time, so you are lying down with your legs extended.

Body check: Make sure both shoulders stay on the floor. You might also place a cushion under your knees if they don't come all the way down to the floor.

Gentle alternative: Lie on your back with your arms around your midsection. Lower knees from side to side, gently and slowly. Take time to move into the twist.

Repetitions: Once on each side

Turn over onto your right side, push down on your left palm and come to a seated position to prepare for supported bound angle.

Supported Bound Angle (Supta Baddha Konasana)

This is a terrific position for quick rejuvenation. The pose opens the hip and groin area, encouraging blood flow. It helps alleviate

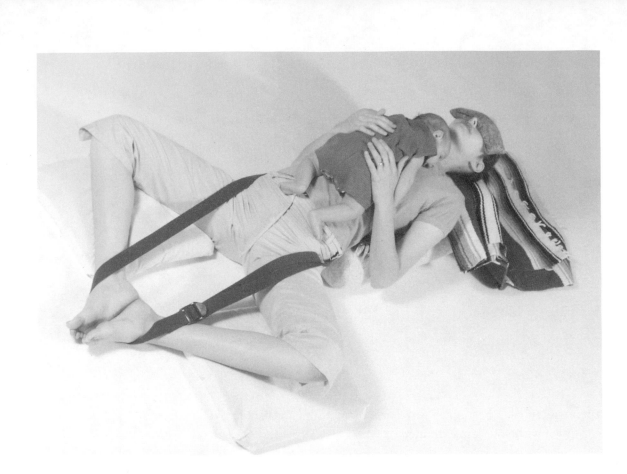

backaches. It also opens up the chest, which is great for new moms because you may feel as if your shoulders are really slumped forward. Hold as long as you want.

Medical cautions: Do not do this pose if you have any nerve problems in your neck or spinal disk conditions.

Where's Baby: You can put your baby right on your chest and place your arms around her.

 ROUTINE 2 (APPROXIMATELY 20 MINUTES BUT DON'T RUSH THROUGH THIS)

Sit comfortably or lie down to begin with a breathing practice.

Three-Part Breath
(Deergha Swaasam)

Do this for eight breaths.

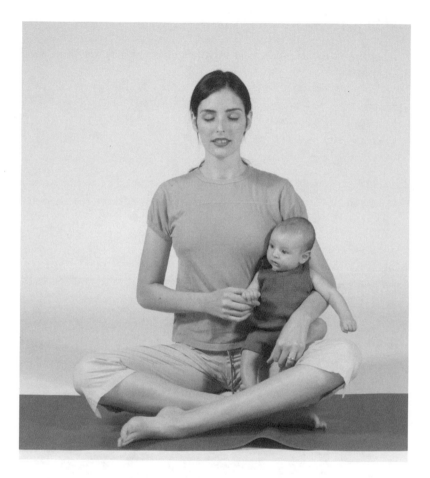

Seated comfortably, move into half neck rolls.

Half Neck Rolls

With your baby next to you or on your lap, do two or more times on each side.

Shoulder Rolls

Shoulder rolls open up the chest and upper back and relieve tension in the shoulders. It's a great movement for moms who hold their baby in a front carrier. You can do these whenever you feel the need.

With your baby next to you or in your lap, do at least three in each direction.

Foot Stretch

This stretch loosens your calf muscles, encourages blood circulation in your lower limbs and minimizes swelling in the feet and an-

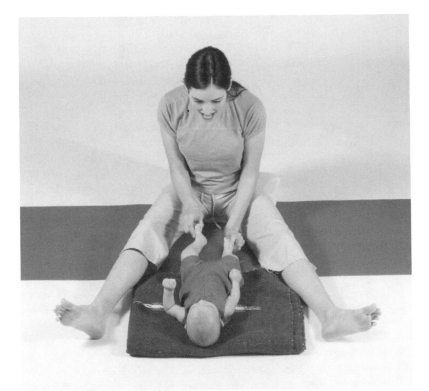

kles. Foot stretches are very important to do if you are confined to bed after a C-section.

Where's Baby: Hold your baby or rest her in your lap. As you wiggle your toes, you can wiggle hers, as well as rotate her ankles gently and play games with her toes.

To begin: Give all your toes a nice wiggle. Rotate your ankles gently to the right, making a slow clockwise circle. Now rotate in the other direction. Do five circles in each direction.

Next, flex your feet, stretching your heels away from you as you point your toes toward yourself. Hold for several seconds and release. Do this flex exercise for about one minute.

Now stand up and stretch your toes like duck feet, imagining webs between them. Lift your toes off the floor and then return them to the floor, two to three times for each foot.

Body check: Make sure your whole body is comfortable as you do these. We tend to neglect the feet, so take some time with this stretch.

Don't be surprised if your feet are bigger after pregnancy. Pregnancy also tends to flatten out feet. In standing poses you can lift your toes off the floor during a stretch—this will create an arch.

Repetitions: Stretch both feet for about one minute per foot. Do foot circles five times in each direction or as often as you desire.

Kegels

Do kegels in child's pose, sitting, or standing, whichever position you find most comfortable.

Lie down on your back.

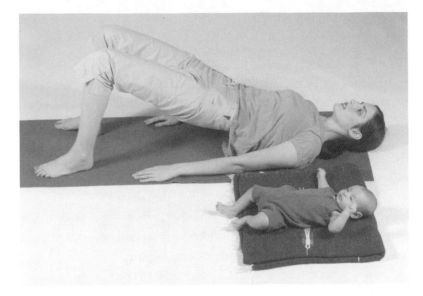

The Bridge

Hold this pose as long as you like.

Staying on your back, move into abdominal work.

Abdominal Work I

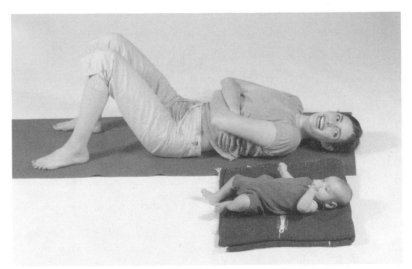

Do at least five of these.

Abdominal Work II

Here is another set of ab exercises.

Where's Baby: Lying beside you

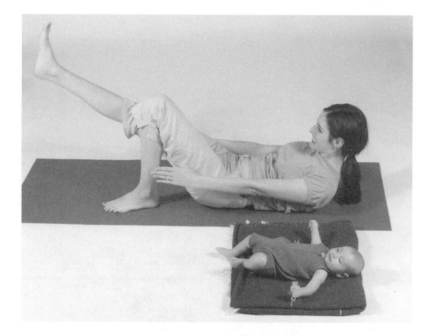

To begin: Lie on the floor (or bed) with your knees bent and the soles of your feet on the floor. Stretch out your arms alongside your body with your palms facing each other. Bring your head and neck off the floor. Extend and raise your right leg. Do five slow leg lifts with your right leg. Don't bring your right leg any higher than the left knee, and try not to let your leg touch the floor between lifts. After five leg lifts, bend your right knee and place the sole of your foot on the floor. Then release your head to the floor. Repeat on the left side.

Body check: Make sure you keep your abdominal muscles engaged as you raise your leg. Do this movement slowly.

Repetitions: Five to ten times, working up to twenty repetitions

C-Sections: Please don't do this version; stay with Abdominal Work I instead. Cross your arms over your midsection to direct the abdominal recti (straight muscles) together as you do the single leg lifts.

Stay on your back.

Knees-to-Chest Rocker

This movement massages your lower-back muscles to relieve tightness and tension.

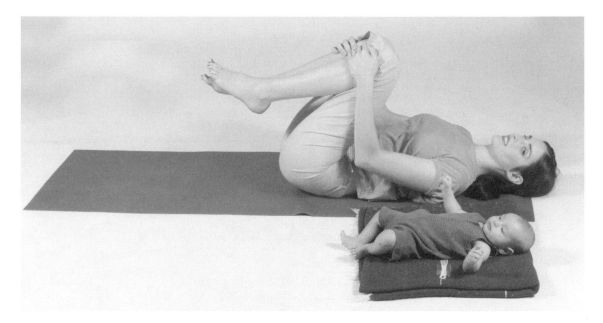

Where's Baby: Lying at your side

To begin: Lie on your back, legs and arms straight. Bring your knees up to your chest and wrap your arms around your legs so you are rolled into a ball. As you feel your lower back opening up, rock gently from side to side, giving your back a massage. Next rock front to back, massaging your spine. Slowly bring your hands away and lower your arms and legs to the floor.

Body check: Enjoy!

Repetitions: Rock as long as it feels good.

Stay on your back to move into baby crocodile spinal twist.

Baby Crocodile Spinal Twist

Do one twist to each side.

Then get pillows and blankets to rest.

Supported Bound Angle (Supta Baddha Konasana)

Hold for as long as you like.

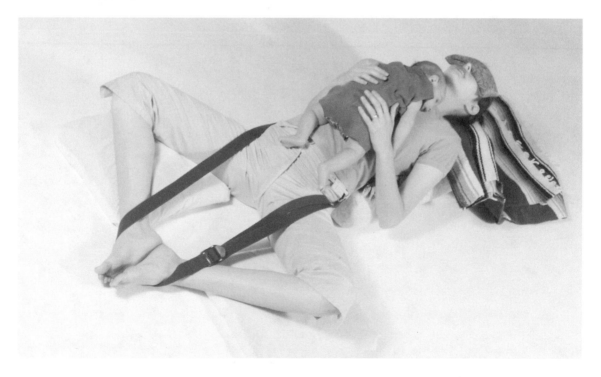

Baby Moves

Your baby is already part of your yoga practice as you hold and touch him during your various poses. But I want to share some poses in which your baby is the main mover. This can be playtime with your baby as you guide him through the gentle movements. These postures will keep him flexible and strengthen his muscles. Watch his response: babies love the motion and your touch during the following baby asanas, and it's fun to see the smiles on his face. This is a lovely way to bond. When your baby starts crawling he will still enjoy the postures; if he is not interested he will simply crawl away, which might be a good time for you to get in a few yoga postures on your own.

Here are some pointers as you start these baby postures now and continue them through your baby's first year:

- Always follow your baby's cue; he will let you know if he likes the movements by laughing and smiling. Likewise, if your baby doesn't like them, he will let you know.

- Do all motions gently; do not force movements. Do not do these postures right after your baby has eaten.

- Please wait to do these baby postures until your baby is about three weeks old. While he is a newborn, keep him swaddled and cozy and practice with him close by. (New babies like to be swaddled—after all, they have been in the uterus for nine months. Watch as your newborn pulls in his arms because he is used to hitting the uterine wall.) Once he has adjusted to the wider range of motion outside the womb, you can begin these movements.

BABY BICYCLES

Baby bicycles help a baby's coordination, keep her limber, and strengthen the legs. This movement can also relieve constipation and help with gas and colic.

Where's Baby: Lying down on her back on a blanket

"It's a new frontier being a mom, and doing yoga with Madeline is very centering and healing. I do stretching with her, and she knows the breathing and is entertained by it. They model a lot from us, and this includes calmness and relaxation. Chanting has become her lullaby. It's such a positive thing in our lives, emotionally, physically and spiritually."

—BRENDA AND
DAUGHTER MADELINE

To begin: As baby lies on her back, hold her right foot and bend her right knee. Her left leg stays on the floor. Then do the same with the left leg and foot. Repeat, alternating between legs, several times. Then hold her feet gently and move them slowly in a circle, as if she is cycling. As you do this, blow gently on her soles.

Repetitions: Bend each knee several times.

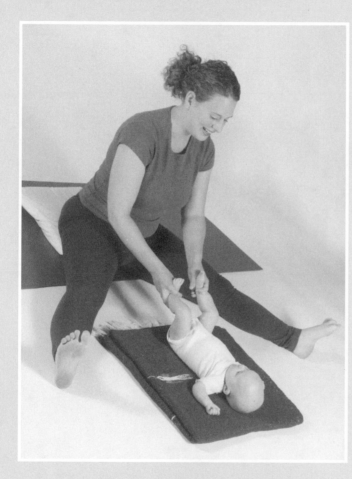

"The weight is outside, not in your belly anymore. It goes beyond the exercise—the bond is really important, and it's really fun, too. It's important for the baby to have pleasurable experiences. Especially early on, the baby can't move by himself, so you help him; it benefits his development. And it gives me the confidence to do all sorts of things with Nathanael, to carry him around in many different ways and to hold him upside down. We used it for exercise and for playing. I showed the yoga to my mother and she liked to do it with him; it was a good way for her to relate to him right away."

—TAMAR AND SON NATHANAEL

BABY BOW POSE

The baby bow pose, which you can start when your baby is three weeks old, strengthens your baby's leg muscles.

Where's Baby: Lying on her belly on a blanket

To begin: With your baby on her belly, hold her right leg. Now bend her right knee, bringing her right heel toward her buttocks. Repeat with her left leg. Then repeat moving both legs together.

Repetitions: Three times with each leg separately and three times with both legs together

HOW BIG IS BABY?

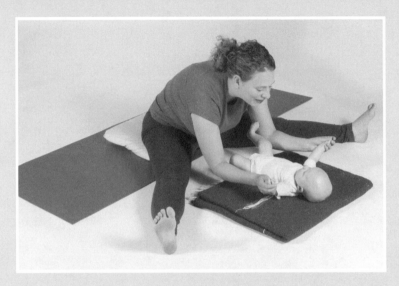

This movement, which you can start when your baby is four weeks old, develops your baby's upper-body strength and motor coordination.

Where's Baby: Lying down on her back on a blanket

To begin: Open your baby's arms so they are in line with her shoulders. Ask your baby: "How big is Baby?" Bring your baby's arms up above her chest, touching her hands together. Lower your baby's arms back down to the floor.

Repetitions: Three times

Begin sitting.

Cleansing Breath

This breathing practice is terrific for releasing tension.

Where's Baby: In front of you or in your lap

To begin: Inhale through your nose with your mouth closed. Exhale through an open mouth, ahhhh!

You can also add movement as you do the cleansing breath. Stand up and open your legs to a comfortable position. As you inhale, lift your arms over your head. As you exhale, bend your knees, bringing your arms down. If your baby is lying in front of you, make contact with her as you lower your arms.

Yawning during this breathing practice is normal; your body is experiencing the benefits of bringing more oxygen in and it wants even more, so you yawn.

Body check: Relax and let go.

Repetitions: Three times. Practice whenever you feel the need, with or without movement.

Sitting or standing, whichever position is most comfortable, move into half neck rolls.

Half Neck Rolls

Do three half neck rolls to each side.

Shoulder Rolls

Do three shoulder rolls.

Come onto your hands and knees for cat and cow.

After Your Baby Is Born

Cat and Cow

Cat and cow pose stretches your back and strengthens your abdominal muscles. This relaxing and energizing movement is great for relieving lower-back aches.

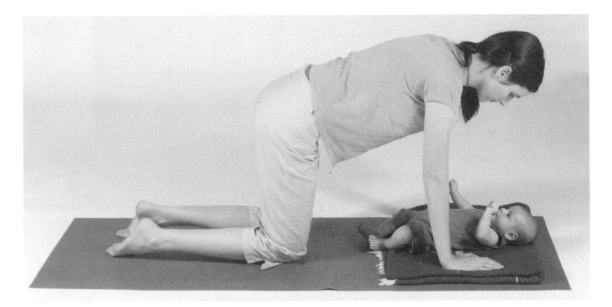

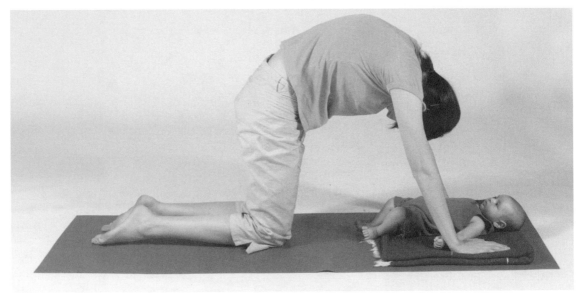

Where's Baby: Lying in front of you. When you bring your head down, smile at her and wiggle your hair on her tummy. You can also shake your head from side to side, letting your hair fly—your baby will enjoy this.

To begin: Get on the floor on your hands and knees. Form a tabletop, with your hands under your shoulders and your knees below your hips; do not lock your elbows. Inhale. As you exhale, move your pelvis slightly back and down, bringing energy through your spine.

Now let your head hang down so you are looking at your knees. Use your abdominals here; bring your belly button in toward your spine. Inhale, bringing your pelvis slightly forward as you lengthen your spine and gently look up. Exhale and repeat.

Body check: Do not create big arches or curves in your spine; you are lengthening the spine by moving your buttocks and pelvis backward and down, and forward and up.

Repetitions: Three times

Child's Pose

Child's pose provides a great stretch for the spine in addition to relaxing your entire body and mind.

Where's Baby: Lying in front of you. When you come down, wiggle your head to tickle your baby with your hair or give your baby a "raspberry" on her belly.

To begin: From your hands and knees, open your knees a little wider, bringing your toes together and your heels apart. Move your buttocks back to rest between your heels, and bring your forehead down toward the floor. Breathe and relax. You can keep your arms crossed under your forehead, stretched straight above your head or stretched out back along your body—whichever you find most comfortable. Rest in child's pose as long as you need to feel the tension dissolve from your body and your mind quieting. Concentrate on slow, rhythmic breathing.

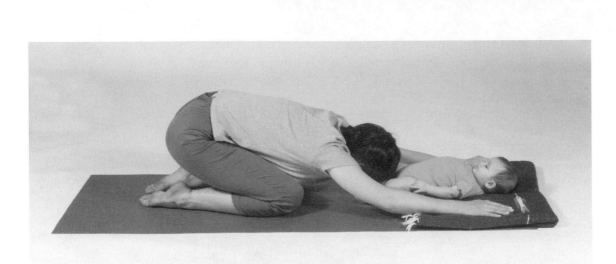

When you are ready, walk your hands up to your chest and inhale into a sitting position. Or, from your hands and knees, come onto your knees, bring one foot to the floor, curl back the toes of your back leg and come up to standing.

Body check: Be aware of being comfortable; use blankets or pillows under your knees or chest if desired.

Repetitions: Once, twice or as many times as you need throughout the day. This is a great posture on its own. It's a great back stretch and also a great position in which to do your kegels.

Come to standing to move into pelvic rolls.

Standing Pelvic Rolls

Standing pelvic rolls tone and strengthen your pelvic and abdominal muscles. They also relieve lower-back aches.

Where's Baby: Hold your baby facing into your chest. Support her from underneath her buttocks; this is her center of gravity.

To begin: Holding your baby facing in, let your arms and shoulders relax. Allow your baby's weight to bring your shoulders down, but don't collapse your upper body; keep your chest open. Move your legs a little more than hip width apart, knees slightly bent. Begin a rotation by stretching out with your right hip, extending your buttocks back, stretching with your left hip, then gently coming forward. As you do rotations, let your baby lean against you, joining you in this motion. It's a fun ride!

Body check: Try big circles and little circles; see which feels better. Keep your knees slightly bent. Check your posture. Move your hips, not your shoulders. It's fun to do these to music.

Repetitions: Three times in each direction

From standing, lie down.

The Wave

The wave is a great massage for the spine.

Where's Baby: On a blanket close by

To begin: Lie on your back. As you inhale, raise your hips off the floor and bring your arms overhead. As you exhale, lower your hips and bring your arms down along the sides of your body.

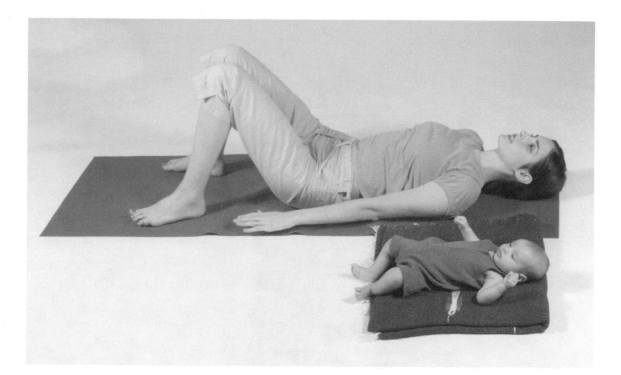

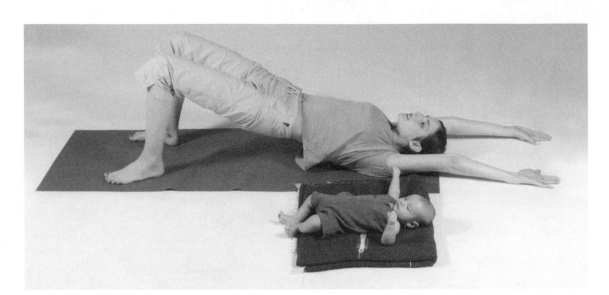

Body check: Relax and enjoy this nice massage of your spine.

Repetitions: Three times

Stay on your back.

Knees-to-Chest Rocker

Do five rocks from side to side and front and back, or as many as your body asks for.

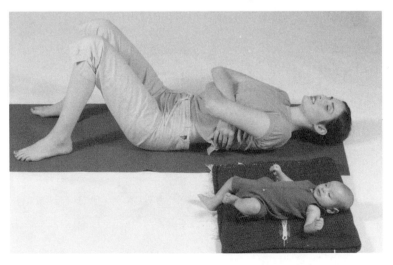

Abdominal Work I

Do five repetitions of this ab exercise.

Relax your abs by moving into:

Baby Crocodile
Spinal Twist

Hold the twist as long as you like on each side.

Now it's time to relax.

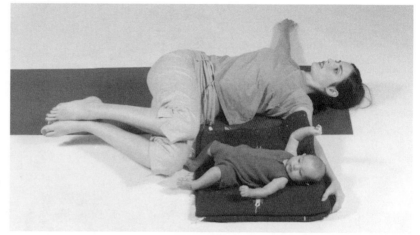

Savasana

This posture helps bring deep relaxation to your entire body while quieting the mind. It is a good position to do with three-part breath. Hold as long as you want.

Where's Baby: Next to you

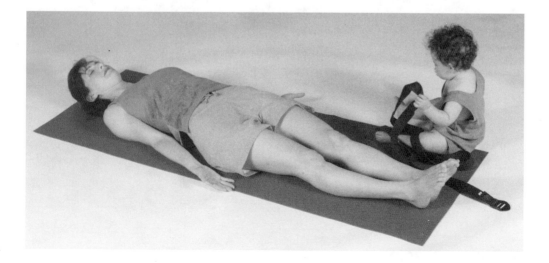

Begin in a seated position (cross-legged if it is comfortable for you).

Belly Breathing

Practicing belly breathing strengthens your abdominal muscles. It also focuses the mind, balancing mind, body and soul.

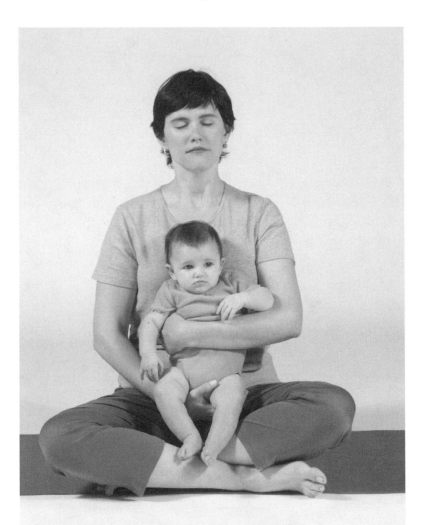

Kapaalabhaati (Deep Diaphragm Breathing)

This warming, energetic breath tones the abdominal muscles and gives the internal organs a massage. Begin this practice right after birth, but not with a forceful exhalation. After you've done six weeks of Kapaalabhaati, your exhalation can increase in force.

Medical caution: Never do this breathing during pregnancy.

Repetitions: Three rounds, working up to twenty breaths each round

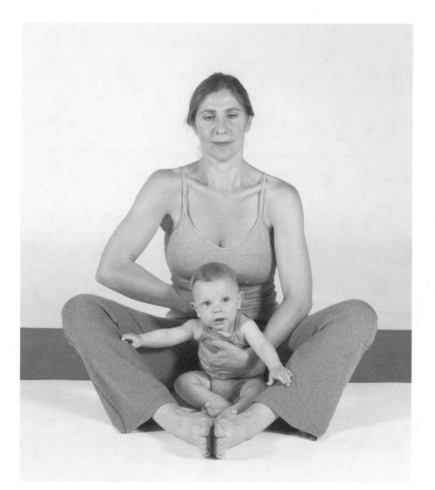

Half Neck Rolls

Do three half neck rolls.

Shoulder Rolls

Do three shoulder rolls.

Come onto your hands and knees.

Wag the Tail

This movement gives a good stretch to the muscles between the ribs.

Where's Baby: Lying in front of you on a blanket

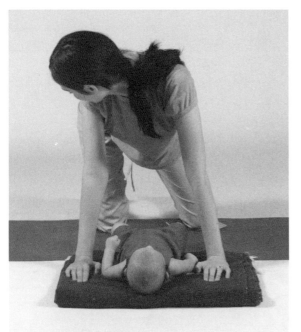

To begin: Come onto your hands and knees. Position your palms under your shoulders and your knees under your hips. Lift your belly button up toward your spine. Contracting your abdominal muscles, inhale. As you exhale, look over your right shoulder as you push out your right hip, bringing your right shoulder and right hip toward each other. Inhale back to center. Move your head from side to side, letting your baby grab your hair. Then repeat on the other side.

Body check: Contract your abdominal muscles as you do this pose.

Repetitions: Three times on each side

Stay on your hands and knees.

Cat and Cow

Do three flows of this movement, or you can do more if your body asks for more.

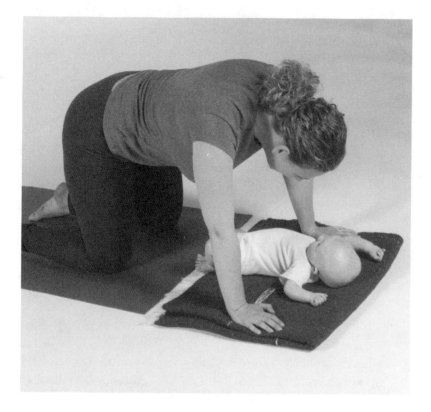

Downward Dog

This is a terrific stretching movement for the back and hamstrings. Downward dog also strengthens the upper body and tones your abdominals.

Where's Baby: Lying in front of you

To begin: Begin on your hands and knees. Make sure to open up between your fingers. Curl your toes underneath. Inhale, exhale and push up, moving your buttocks toward the ceiling in an in-

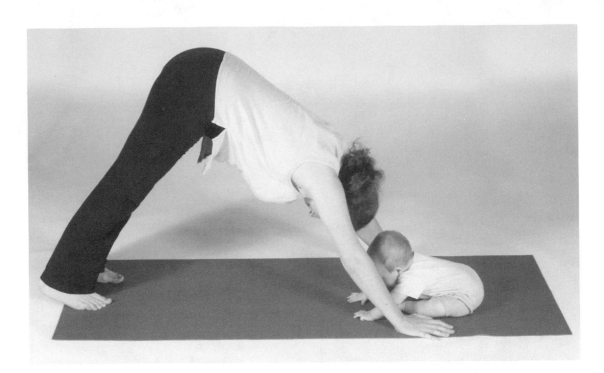

verted V. Bring your belly button toward the spine and bring your heels down toward the floor. Open up between your shoulder blades, let your head relax and look at your knees.

Time: Stay in this position for at least three breaths.

Walk the dog variation: While in downward dog, raise your left heel, bending the knee. Now bring the right heel down toward the floor and hold for ten seconds. Raise your right heel and bring your left heel to the floor, holding for ten seconds. Finish by bringing both heels back down toward the floor.

Body check: Be aware of the feet and legs; they should be close together. Let the shoulders relax. Make sure not to lock your elbows (hyperextension weakens the ligaments).

Repetitions: Do once.

Come down onto your hands and knees to move into:

Yoga Mom,
Buddha Baby

Child's Pose

Relax into the pose for at least three breaths.

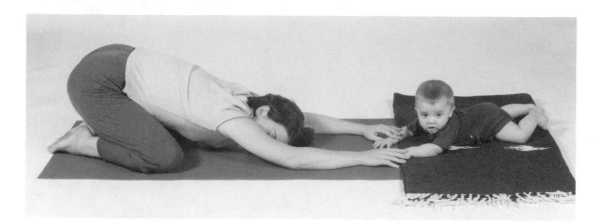

Lift yourself into a seated position. Stretch your legs out in front of you. Inhale, exhale and slowly lower yourself down into a lying position, using your abdominals.

Total Lying Stretch

You will stretch in two directions at once to stretch your entire body.

Where's Baby: Close to you

To begin: Lie on your back, stretching your arms overhead. Inhale. Feel as though you're reaching in two directions. Press the small of your back into the floor. Exhale and release. Relax.

Body check: Enjoy; relax.

Repetitions: Three times

Bend your knees, with the soles of your feet on the floor.

Abdominal Work II

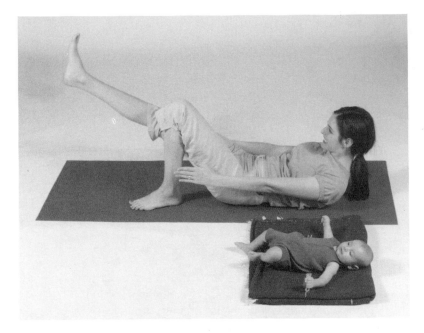

Do ten leg lifts on each side.

Knees-to-Chest Rocker

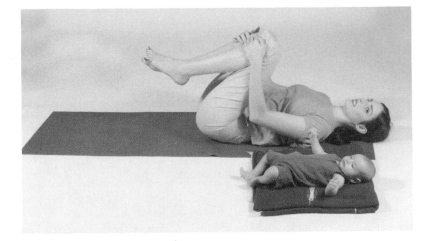

Rock back and forth and side to side.

Baby Crocodile
Spinal Twist

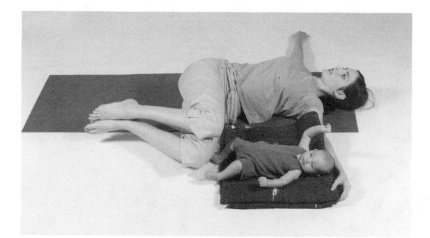

Hold the twist on each side for as long as you like.

Get your props to move into the final relaxation pose.

Supported Reclining Pose

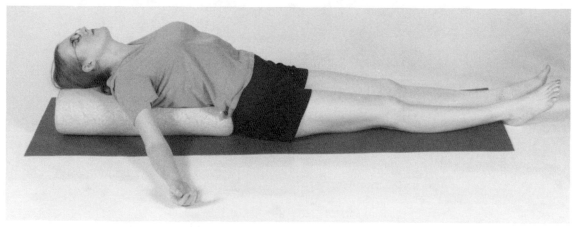

This very calming position opens up the chest and helps respiration. Hold as long as you like.

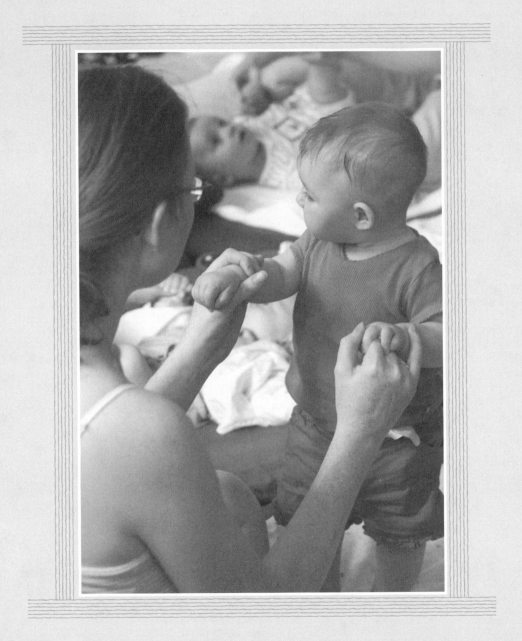

Nine

Six to Twelve Weeks

Yay! You've made it to six weeks. (I always say the first three weeks are a blur.) Now your uterus has returned to its normal size and by this time your breasts probably won't feel as heavy as they did those first few weeks after you gave birth. Hopefully, you have slowly come to a settled "I can handle this" phase, although you're exhausted and sleep-deprived and can't remember anything. But do remember it's important to look after yourself too.

This is a great time to find a class for you and your baby or a mother's group. Long days with a baby can feel isolating. It's usually at this point that moms start coming to my postpartum class. Many women tell me they have been trying to come to class for weeks but they just don't seem to make it; new motherhood takes time to get used to. My daughter Rachel won't like my telling this story, but I remember being ready to walk out the door and hearing an explosion of poop. I knew I wasn't going anywhere soon. Motherhood teaches you flexibility—you just have to go with the flow.

When you do make it out of the house, you will be carrying a diaper bag and other paraphernalia. Plus, your baby will weigh more than she did, not only making her harder to hold over long periods of time but also presenting a phenomenon witnessed only by new mothers: nature's ultimate progressive weight system. This makes practicing yoga that much more important. Holding your growing baby as you practice will help you to increase muscle tone and strength. It will also encourage correct posture.

At this time your baby will start giving you smiles; it's beautiful to watch a baby smile with mom as mom does her yoga. Touch is very important to him—it is stimulating and reassuring as he expands the boundaries of his senses. During this time, remember not to be overcritical of yourself. Everything takes time, including confidence in your yoga and your motherhood.

Routines from Six to Twelve Weeks

ROUTINE 1 (APPROXIMATELY 20 MINUTES)

Begin in a seated position (cross-legged if it is comfortable for you).

Forward Neck Release

This movement releases tension in your neck, shoulders and upper back. It also provides a nice stretch for the vertebrae in the cervical spine.

Do the entire sequence two or three times.

Stretch your legs in front of you.

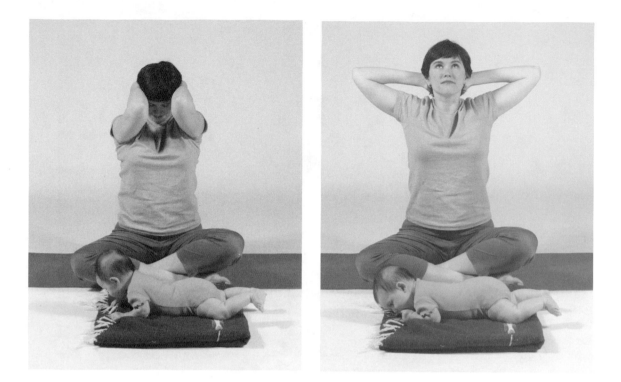

Foot Stretch

This stretch loosens your calf muscles, encourages blood circulation in your lower limbs and minimizes swelling in the feet and ankles.

Where's Baby: Hold your baby or rest her in your lap. As you wiggle your toes, you can wiggle hers, as well as rotate her ankles gently and play games with her toes.

To begin: Give all your toes a nice wiggle. Rotate your ankles gently to the right, making a slow clockwise circle. Now rotate in the other direction. Do five circles in each direction.

Next, flex your feet, stretching your heels away from you as you point your toes toward yourself. Hold for several seconds and release. Do this flex exercise for one minute.

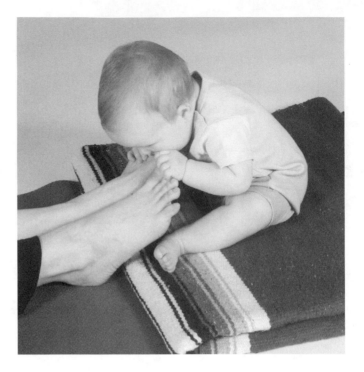

Now stand up and stretch your toes like duck feet, imagining webs between your toes. Lift your toes off the floor and then return them to the floor, two to three times for each foot.

Body check: Make sure your whole body is comfortable as you do these. We tend to neglect the feet, so take some time with this stretch.

Pregnancy tends to flatten out feet. In standing poses you can lift your toes off the floor during a stretch; this will create an arch.

Repetitions: Stretch both feet for about one minute per foot. Do foot circles five times in each direction or as often as you desire.

Come onto your hands and knees.

Wag the Tail

This movement gives a good stretch to the muscles between the ribs.

Where's Baby: Lying in front of you on a blanket

To begin: Come onto your hands and knees. Position your palms under your shoulders and your knees under your hips. Lift your belly button up toward your spine. Contracting your abdominal muscles, inhale. As you exhale, look over your right shoulder as you push out your right hip, bringing your right shoulder and right hip toward each other. Inhale back to center. Move your head from side to side, letting your baby grab your hair. Then repeat on the other side.

Body check: Contract your abdominal muscles as you do this pose.

Repetitions: Three times on each side

Stay on your hands and knees.

Cat and Cow

Cat and cow pose stretches your back and strengthens your abdominal muscles. This relaxing and energizing movement is great for relieving aches in the lower back.

Where's Baby: Lying in front of you. When you bring your head down, smile at your baby and wiggle your hair on her tummy. You can shake your head from side to side, letting your hair fly—your baby will enjoy this.

To begin: Get on the floor on your hands and knees. Form a tabletop, with your hands under your shoulders and your knees below your hips; do not lock your elbows. Inhale. As you exhale, move your pelvis slightly back and down, bringing energy through your spine.

Now let your head hang down so you are looking at your knees. Use your abdominals here; bring your belly button in toward your spine. Inhale, bringing your pelvis slightly forward as you lengthen your spine and lift your head gently looking up. Exhale and repeat.

I'm trying to find different ways of incorporating my new life and my body, and yoga allows me to combine things. I feel a little bit taller, and Liliana always has a good night's sleep after we do yoga.

—KASIA AND DAUGHTER LILIANA

Six to Twelve Weeks

Body check: Do not create big arches or curves in your spine; you are lengthening the spine by moving your buttocks and pelvis backward and down, and forward and up, not arching your back.

Repetitions: Several times

Child's Pose

Child's pose provides a great stretch for the spine, in addition to relaxing your entire body and mind.

Where's Baby: Lying in front of you. When you come down, wiggle your head to tickle your baby with your hair or give your baby a "raspberry" on her belly.

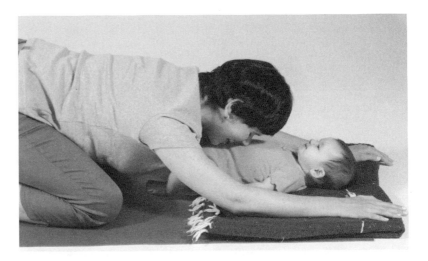

To begin: From your hands and knees, open your knees a little wider, bringing your toes together and heels apart. Move your buttocks back to rest between your heels, and bring your forehead down toward the floor. Breathe and relax. You can keep your arms crossed under your forehead, stretched straight above your head or stretched out back along your body—whichever you find most comfortable. Rest in child's pose as long as you need to feel the tension dissolve from your body and your mind quieting. Concentrate on slow, rhythmic breathing.

Body check: Be aware of being comfortable; use blankets or pillows under your knees or chest if desired.

Repetitions: Once, twice or as many times as you need throughout the day. This is a great posture on its own. It's a great back stretch and also a great position in which to do your kegels.

Stand up slowly by coming into diamond pose (see page 71). Pick up your baby. Bring one leg forward and come up to standing.

Flying Babies

This slow, gentle motion soothes and entertains your baby while it builds strength in your arms, back and chest.

Do slow, gentle motions with your baby.

Where's Baby: At six weeks, hold your baby facing toward you. At twelve weeks, baby can face out.

To begin: Part one: Stand with your feet a comfortable distance apart. Hold your baby against your chest (facing outward), with one or both hands under her buttocks. Inhale, exhale and lift your baby to the right as you bring your weight to the right side. Your knees will bend and then straighten when your baby is all the way over to the right. Reverse and "fly" your baby to the left side. This should be a slow, gentle movement.

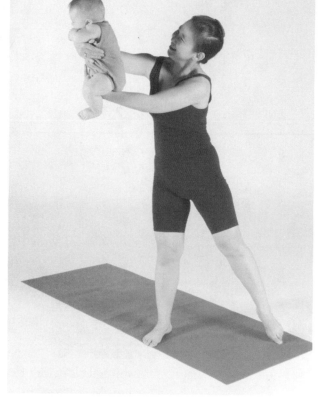

Body check: Let your shoulders relax. Put on some favorite music and, as always, check your posture, breathe and enjoy.

Baby check: Make sure your baby is enjoying the motion; base whether to quicken the pace or slow it down upon your baby's reaction.

Six to Twelve Weeks

Repetitions: A few times on each side

Stay standing to move into pelvic rolls.

Standing Pelvic Rolls

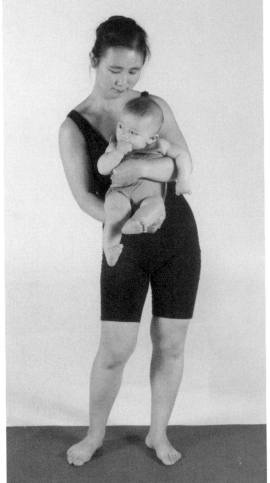

Standing pelvic rolls tone and strengthen your pelvic and abdominal muscles. They also relieve lower-back aches.

Where's Baby: For a baby under eight weeks, hold her facing into your chest; for one older than eight weeks, hold her facing out, resting her back against your belly and chest. Put one arm under her buttocks and the other around her belly. Or you can use both arms to make a circle, with your baby sitting inside. Support your baby from underneath her buttocks; this is her center of gravity.

To begin: Holding your baby in or out depending on her age, let your arms and shoulders relax. Allow your baby's weight to relax your shoulders down, but don't collapse your upper body. Move your legs a little more than hip width apart, knees slightly bent. Begin a rotation by stretching out with your right hip, extending the buttocks back, stretching with your left hip, then gently thrusting forward. As you do rotations, let your baby lean against you, joining you in this motion. It's a fun ride!

Body check: Try big circles and little circles; see which feels better. Keep your knees slightly bent. Check your posture. Move your hips, not your shoulders. It's fun to do these to music.

Yoga Mom,
Buddha Baby

Repetitions: Three times in each direction

From standing, lie down to move into abdominal work.

134

Abdominal Work I

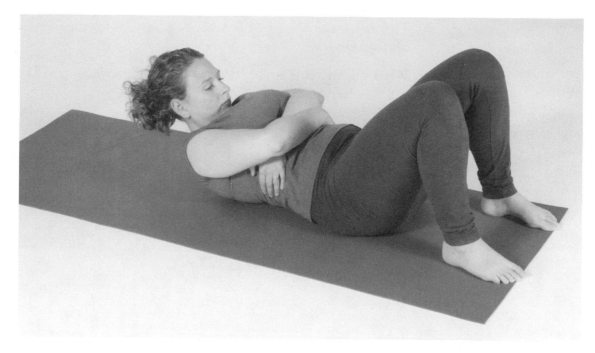

This exercise tones and strengthens the abdominal muscles. You can do it on the floor or in bed.

Where's Baby: Resting against your thighs or lying next to you

To begin: Lie down on your back. Bend your knees, keeping the soles of your feet on the floor. Cross your arms over your midsection and exhale. Contract your abdominals by bringing the belly button back to the spine and raise your head and neck off the floor. Lower yourself back down again.

Body check: While doing this movement, it is important to focus on the abs; visualize them working. Do not use your neck or other muscles to raise or lower yourself.

Repetitions: Begin with five and work up to fifteen to twenty or whatever is comfortable per day.

Stay on your back.

Six to Twelve Weeks

Knees-to-Chest Rocker

This movement massages your lower-back muscles to relieve tightness and tension.

Where's Baby: Lying at your side or on your shins facing you. She will like the ride.

To begin: Lie on your back, your legs and arms straight. Bring your knees up to your chest and wrap your arms around your legs so you are rolled into a ball. As you feel your lower back opening up, rock gently from side to side, giving your back a massage. Next rock front to back, massaging your spine. Slowly bring your hands away and lower your arms and legs to the floor.

Body check: Enjoy!

Repetitions: Rock as long as it feels good.

Sit up.

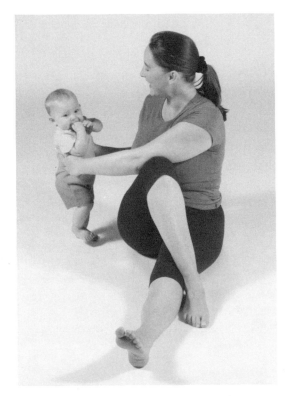

Half Spinal Twist (Ardha Matsyendrasana)

This pose tones the abdominal area; it stretches the back and side muscles, helps with digestive problems, keeps the spine flexible, squeezes toxins out of the spine as if one is "wringing a washcloth," and massages internal organs.

Where's Baby: Close to you or sitting with you; you can move her from side to side as you twist.

To begin: In a seated position, stretch your legs out in front of you. Keep your left leg straight as you cross your right foot over your left knee. Keep sitting up tall. Bring your right hand behind your spine. Bring your left arm to the outside of the right knee. Twist and look over your right shoulder. Breathe comfortably, using your breath to help you twist. Inhale and sit up tall; exhale, letting the breath move you a little farther into the twist. Stay there, holding for three breaths.

To come out of this pose, inhale and bring your head back to center. Exhale and release your arms. Inhale, exhale and look over your left shoulder. Return to center. Repeat on the other side.

Body check: Keep both buttocks on the floor. Check your posture; make sure you have a tall back.

Repetitions: Do once on each side.

Get your props to move into this final relaxation pose.

Supported Bound Angle (Supta Baddha Konasana)

This is a terrific position for quick rejuvenation. The pose opens the hip and groin area, encouraging blood flow. It also helps alleviate backaches. It opens up the chest, which is great for moms because you may feel as if your shoulders are really slumped forward. Hold as long as you want.

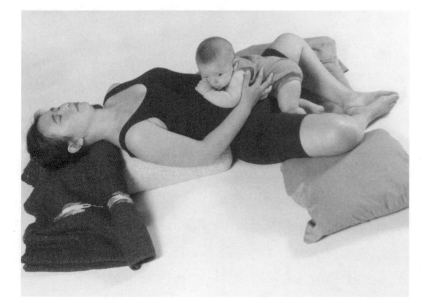

Medical cautions: Do not do this pose if you have any nerve problems in your neck or spinal disk conditions.

Where's Baby: You can put your baby right on your chest; place your arms around her.

⊰ ROUTINE 2 (APPROXIMATELY 30 MINUTES) ⊱

Begin in a seated position (cross-legged if it is comfortable for you).

Half Neck Rolls

As I'm sure you've noticed, bigger breasts, breast- or bottle-feeding and carrying your baby add tension to the back and neck muscles. Half neck rolls relieve tension in the neck and shoulders. Be aware of

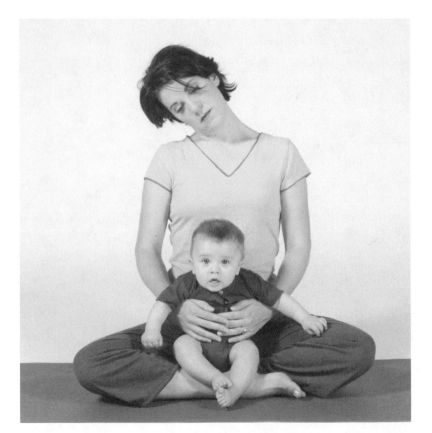

your shoulders and relax them during this movement. If an area feels achy or tight, breathe into that spot to let go of tension. To do that, as you inhale visualize bringing oxygen to the tight area, and as you exhale breathe out the tension. Notice if one side feels tighter than the other; what do you do differently on that side of the body? If you hear cracks or pops, it's just tension being released from the joints.

As you do the neck rolls, you may find that you want to sigh or moan or groan. Please do! This helps relieve tension and makes your jaw and facial muscles relax.

Shoulder Rolls

Shoulder rolls open up the chest and upper back and relieve tension in the shoulders. It's a great movement for moms who hold their baby in a front carrier. You can do these whenever you feel the need. Do at least three circles in each direction.

Come onto your hands and knees.

Child's Pose

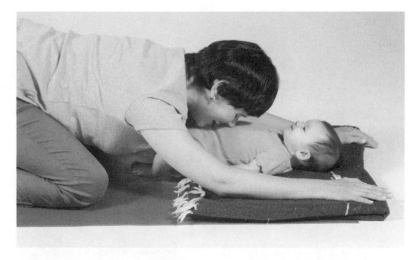

Relax in this pose; it's also a good position in which to practice your kegels.

Downward Dog

This is a terrific stretching movement for the back and hamstrings. It also strengthens the upper body and tones your abdominals.

Where's Baby: Lying in front of you

To begin: Begin on your hands and knees. Make sure to open up between your fingers. Curl your toes underneath. Inhale, exhale and push up, moving your buttocks toward the ceiling in an inverted V. Bring your belly button toward the spine and bring your heels down toward the floor. Open up between your shoulder blades, let your head relax and look at your knees.

Time: Stay in this position for at least three breaths.

Walk the dog variation: While in downward dog, raise your left heel, bending the knee. Now bring the right heel down toward the floor and hold for ten seconds. Raise your right heel and bring your left

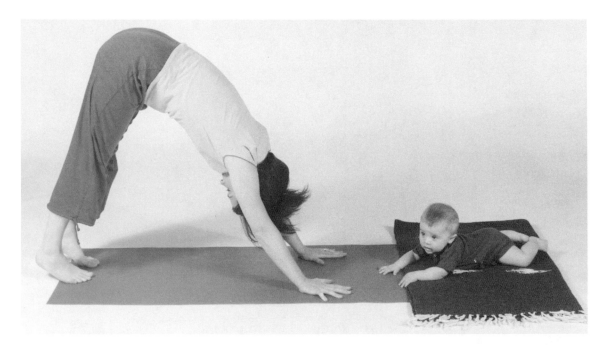

heel to the floor, holding for ten seconds. Finish by bringing both heels back down toward the floor.

Body check: Be aware of the feet and legs; they should be close together. Let the shoulders relax. Make sure not to lock your elbows (hyperextension weakens the ligaments).

Repetitions: Do once, holding for three breaths.

From downward dog, come to your hands and knees, then descend onto your belly.

Cobra

This pose tones and strengthens the upper and lower back and abdominal muscles. It also massages internal organs and opens up the thyroid gland.

Where's Baby: In front of you

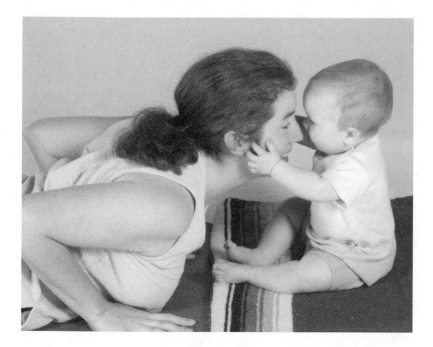

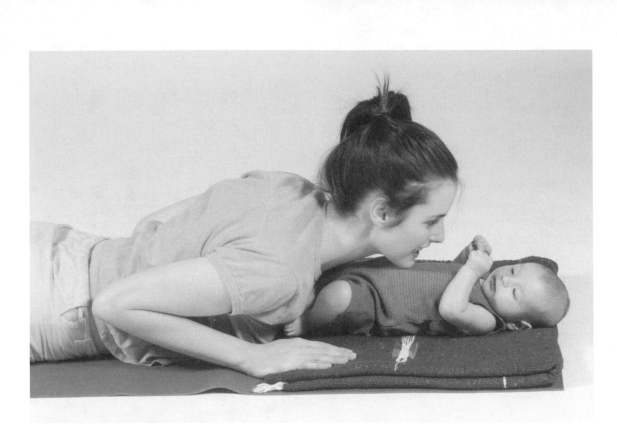

To begin: Lying on your belly, bring your palms underneath your shoulders. Bring your forehead to the floor; make sure your legs and feet are also on the floor. As you inhale, lengthen from the base of your spine and reach out from the crown of the head. Your nose and chin will brush the mat. Using your palms for gentle support, lift your upper body forward and up, opening up through the chest. Keep your shoulders relaxed, elbows slightly bent alongside the body. Lift the belly up to the spine using your abs, but keep your pelvis on the floor. Take three gentle breaths. Slowly lower your back down, vertebra by vertebra, allowing your chin to touch the mat first, and then your forehead. Turn your head to the side. Bring your arms alongside your body and relax. You can also relax into child's pose.

Body check: Keep your pelvis on the floor.

Repetitions: Do once, taking three breaths.

Yoga Mom,
Buddha Baby

Roll onto your back and come into a sitting position.

Side Bends

Side bends are great for stretching your side muscles from the neck down to the pelvis, for opening up the chest and upper back, for realigning the spine and for toning the waist.

Where's Baby: In front of you on a blanket

To begin: Sit comfortably, checking your posture to make sure both buttocks are touching the floor. Interlace your fingers, palms away from you, and stretch your arms out in front. Inhale, lift your arms toward the ceiling, expanding your rib cage, chest and upper back.

Now place your hands behind your head. Bring your elbows out to the sides, stretching your shoulders and opening up your chest. Inhale. On the exhale, bend to the right. Bring your right hand down, palm to the floor, and walk your fingers out. Keep your belly back toward the spine and breathe. Hold the stretch for three breaths, then inhale and come back to center. When you are sitting up straight again, exhale and repeat on the left side.

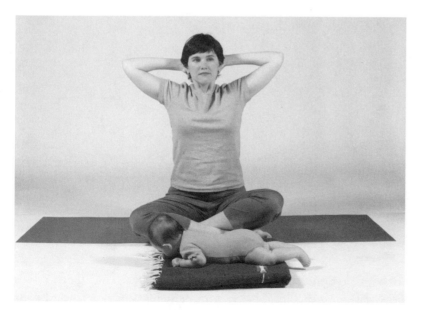

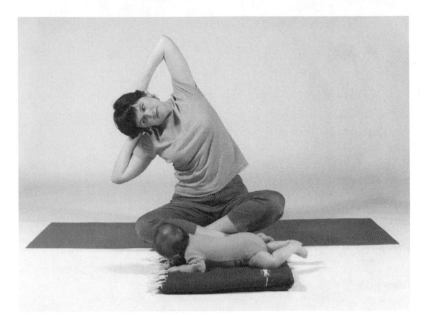

Body check: In order to engage your abdominal muscles, do not pull your belly button in so much that you can't breathe. Instead, just gently contract your abdominal muscles.

Make sure to breathe and relax. This may be easier said than done, so focus on your breathing as you move into a posture. Like now— as you read this, be aware of breathing and relaxing. It helps!

Repetitions: Two to three times to each side

Lie down on your back.

The Bridge

The bridge works the buttocks (gluteus muscle), which helps alleviate stress on the lower back. It also stretches the fronts of the thighs.

Where's Baby: On a blanket in front of you

To begin: Lie on your back and bend your knees, keeping the soles of your feet on the floor. Bring your belly button back toward your spine, squeeze your buttocks and raise your hips off the floor (or bed). In addition to the buttocks, also lift up and contract your pelvic floor muscles. Hold this bridge pose for as long as it feels good. To come down, bring your hands to your sides and lower your hips to the floor.

While in the bridge pose, you can bring your hands into the small of your back to give yourself a nice massage into your kidneys as you support your hips. When you are ready to come out of the position, bring your hands to your sides and lower your hips to the floor (or bed).

Body check: Use your abdominals and glutes.

Repetitions: Do once.

Stay on your back.

Abdominal Work I

Do five to ten times.

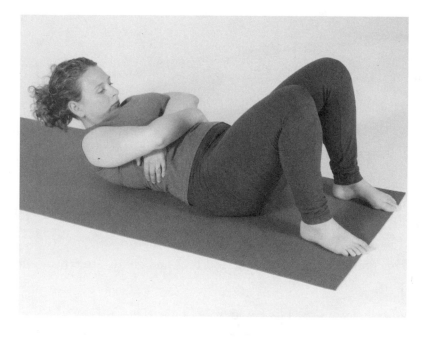

Abdominal Work II

Here is a second set of ab exercises.

Where's Baby: Resting against your thighs, using one or both of your hands to support her. As you lift up your head and upper back, smile for her and play a game of peekaboo.

To begin: Lie on the floor (or bed) with your knees bent and the soles of your feet on the floor. Stretch out your arms alongside your body with your palms facing each other. Bring your head and neck off the floor and your belly button toward the spine. Extend and raise your right leg. Do five slow leg lifts with your right leg. Don't bring your right leg any higher than the left knee. After five leg lifts, bend your right knee and place the sole of your foot on the floor. Then release your head to the floor. Repeat on the left side.

Body check: Make sure you keep your abdominal muscles engaged as you move your leg. Do this movement slowly.

Repetitions: Five to ten times, working up to twenty repetitions

Stay on your back.

Knees-to-Chest Rocker

Rock several times from side to side and front to back.

Lie back down.

Baby Crocodile
Spinal Twist

This posture opens the chest and hips and gently stretches your spine.

Where's Baby: On a blanket in front of you

There is a lot of stress on the body in recovering and carrying around the baby. My body needed more attention than normal. It was a surprise to me to be able to enjoy being with the baby and take care of my body at the same time. I look at yoga as this incredibly efficient use of time. Being with the baby, it feels like the baby is part of the process—[I'm] playing with my baby and also getting exercise and making my body feel better.

—CAROLYN AND
DAUGHTER HANNAH

Yoga Mom,
Buddha Baby

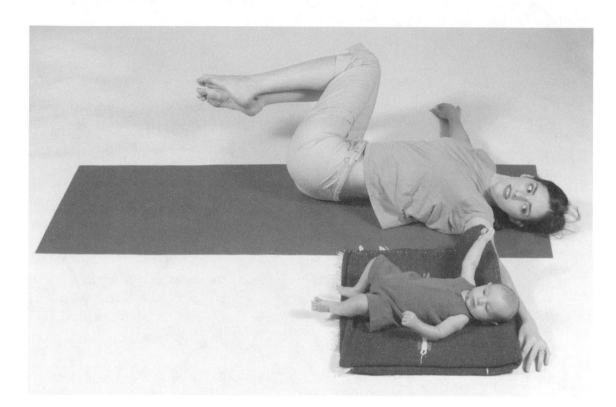

To begin: Lie on your back, with your knees bent to your chest. Extend your arms out to the side, keeping them on the floor perpendicular to your body. Bring both knees together over to the right side of your body and turn your head to the left. Hold this posture as long as you like. Then bring the left knee over to the other side. When your right knee doesn't stay down anymore, bring it over to the left side too. Turn your head to the right. Hold as long as you like. Bring your head and knees back to center, hold, then extend each leg so you are lying down with your legs stretched out.

Body check: Make sure both shoulders stay on the floor. You might also place a cushion under your knees if they don't come all the way down to the floor.

Gentle alternative: Lie on your back with your arms around your midsection. Lower your knees from side to side, gently and slowly. Take time to move into the twist.

Repetitions: Once on each side

Six to Twelve Weeks

Savasana

This posture helps bring deep relaxation to your entire body while quieting the mind. It is a good position to do with three-part breath. Hold as long as you want.

Props: Cushion, pillow or blanket

Where's Baby: Next to you

To begin: Lie down on your back, with a cushion, pillow or rolled-up blanket tucked under your bent knees. Place a small rolled-up blanket under your neck and put a blanket over yourself for warmth, if needed. Breathe fluidly and let your mind and body relax.

Body check: Make any adjustments to your position so that you are comfortable.

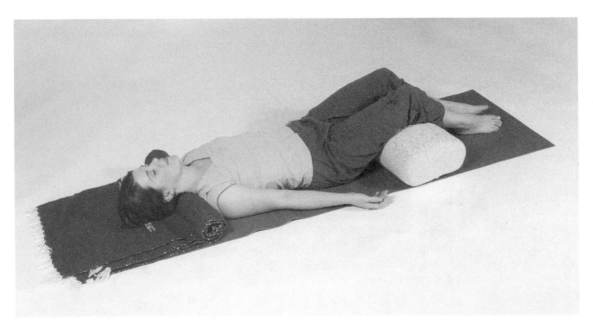

Yoga Mom,
Buddha Baby

Baby Rhymes and Games

I like to have my moms start singing these rhymes and playing these games with their babies when they are six weeks old; that's when your baby is usually ready for more stimulation. When I watch my moms doing these activities with their babies, I notice that everyone is smiling. This is a great way for mom and baby to bond. And the babies especially like the finger play! Always do these movements gently and see if your baby likes them.

OPEN, SHUT THEM

Sit your baby on your lap or put her in front of you lying down. As you sing or chant this song, do the accompanying motions one of two ways. You can do the simple hand motions so your baby watches, or you can hold your baby's hands so she performs the motions. Babies love both doing and watching this!

Open
[Open hands]
Shut them
[Close hands]
Open
[Open hands]
Shut them
[Shut hands]
Put them in your lap, lap, lap
[Hands to lap]
Open
[Open hands]
Shut them
[Close hands]
Open
[Open hands]
Shut them
[Close hands]
Give a little clap, clap, clap
[Clap your hands together or gently clap your hands with your baby's]
Creeping crawling

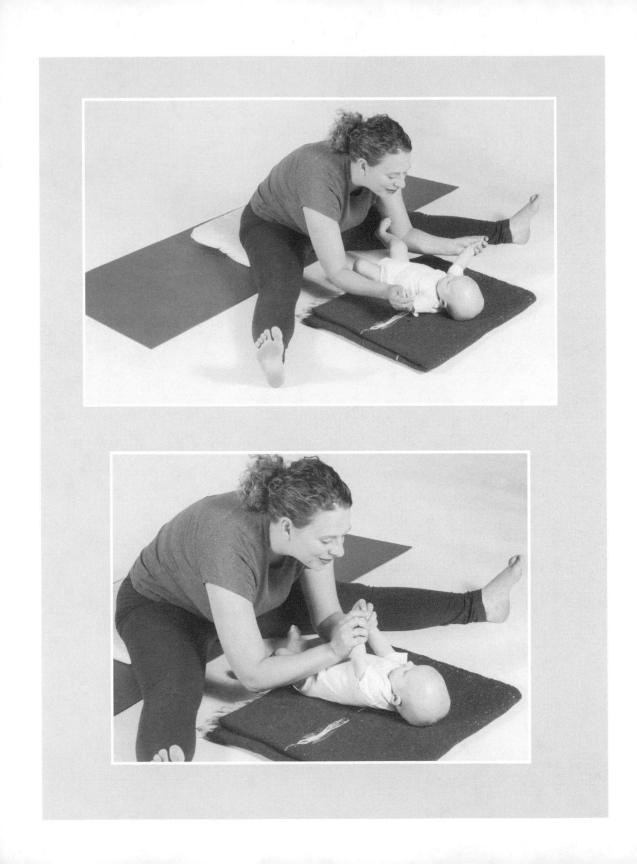

[Crawl your hands up your baby's arms or sides]
Creeping crawling
Up onto your chin, chin, chin
[Crawl your hands up your baby's chin]
Open up your little mouth
[Crawl your hands up to your baby's mouth]
But do not let them in
[Crawl your hands around her cheeks, smile, finish or start again]

ORA'S SONG

I learned this song many years ago from a little girl named Ora (thus the name). Your baby is seated against you, leaning into your belly or against your thigh. Do the motions with your baby's arms as you sing:

Wind, wind, wind them *[Say your baby's name]*
Wind, wind, wind them *[Say your baby's name]*
Pull, pull
Clap, clap, clap
[Repeat!]

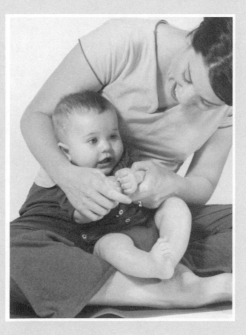

This is fun to sing with babies who can support their own head. Sit on the floor and stretch your legs out, your knees slightly bent. Let your baby ride on top of your thighs. With your legs moving gently up and down, sing to your baby as you move him to the words of the song. I love watching ten or fifteen moms and their babies doing this together in class—it is quite a sight!

The Grand Old Duke of York
He had ten thousand men
He marched them to the top of the hill
[Lift your baby with your arms and bring your knees up, the soles of your feet on the floor]
And he marched them down again
[Bring your baby and your legs down]
And when they were up, they were up
[Lift up baby]
And when they were down, they were down
[Bring baby down]
And when they were only halfway up
[Bring baby halfway up]
They were neither up or down
[Bring baby up and then down]
He marched them to the right
[Bring baby to the right]
He marched them to the left
[Bring baby to the left]
He marched them up the hill again
[Bring baby up]
Oh what a funny sight
[Bring baby down again]
Trot trot to Boston
[Move legs up and down]
Trot trot to Lynn
Trot trot to Gloucester
But don't fall in!
[Open up your legs and let your baby come between them]

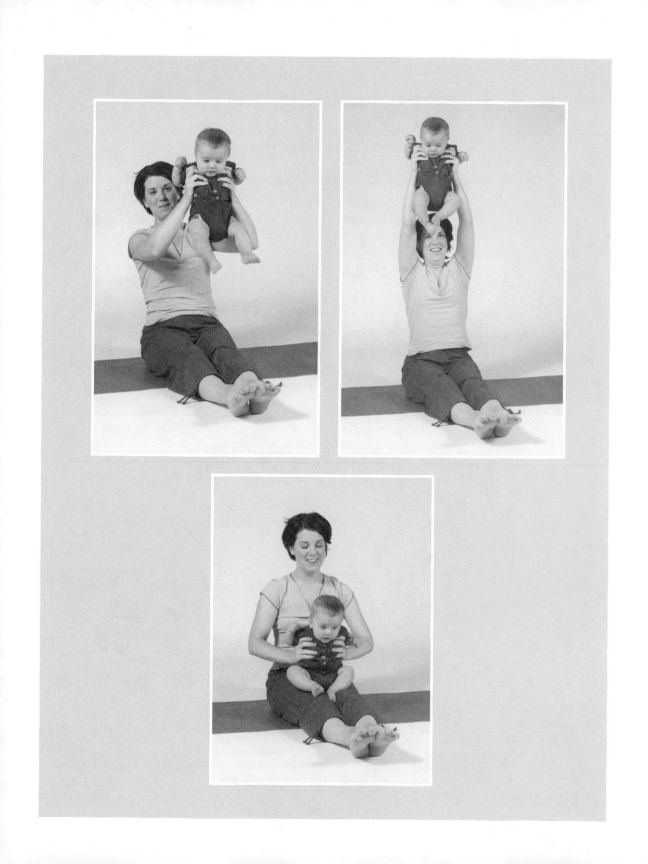

BUMPING UP AND DOWN

This song, popularized by Raffi, and movement are done in the bridge position; your baby rests on your pelvis. Make sure to use your abdominal and gluteal muscles.

Bumping up and down
[Gently move your pelvis up and down (using your gluteal muscles)]
In my little red wagon
Bumping up and down
In my little red wagon
Bumping up and down
In my little red wagon
Won't you be my darling
One wheel's off and the axle's broken
[Gently move your pelvis from side to side. Go to one side, bring your pelvis back to center and move to the other side. Repeat as you sing:]
One wheel's off and the axle's broken
One wheel's off and the axle's broken
Won't you be my darling
(Baby's name) is going to fix it with her hammer
[Gently move your pelvis up and down again]
Baby's going to fix it with her hammer
Baby's going to fix it with her hammer
Won't you be my darling

Alexander loves it. We started when he was seven weeks old. He loves the movement of it; he loves the singing, the clapping, the body manipulation. It has given me more ways to be physical with him.

—ELIZABETH AND SON
ALEXANDER

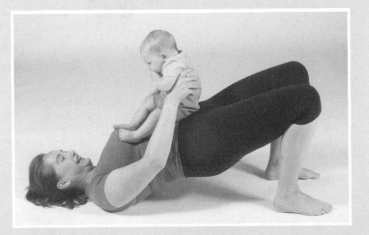

Begin in a standing position.

Cleansing Breath with Movement

You can add body movement as you do your cleansing breath.

Where's Baby: On a blanket in front of you

To begin: Stand with your legs comfortably apart. Inhale deeply through your nose and lift your arms over your head. Exhale through an open mouth, with the sound ahhhh! Bend your knees and bring your arms down.

Body check: Relax and let go.

Repetitions: Do cleansing breath with movement three times. When you are done, stand for a few minutes to notice how you feel.

You can stay standing or move into a comfortable seated position.

Half Neck Rolls

Do three of these.

Shoulder Rolls

Do three of these.

Come onto your hands and knees.

Cat and Cow

Do three of these flowing movements.

Wag the Tail

Stretch to each side three times.

Sit back into child's pose.

Child's Pose

This pose is a great place to do your kegels.

Downward Dog

Hold this for three breaths.

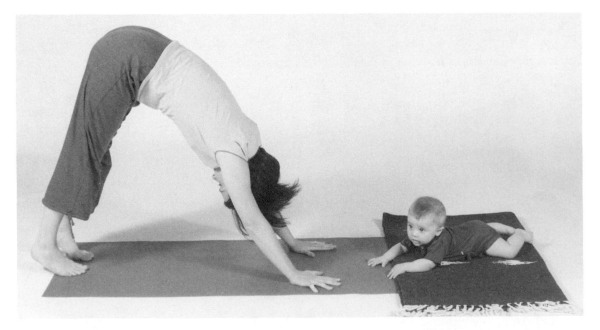

Come back down onto your hands and knees. Sit back into your heels. Sit up on your knees and bring one leg forward. Curl your toes back and stand up.

Flying Babies

Do five to each side; pace your movements on the basis of your baby's enjoyment of flying.

Half Squats with Babies

This movement, using your baby as a "weight," works your arms, thighs and buttocks. As you do this pose, you can say to your baby "Baby goes up-up-up-up-up," then "Baby goes down-down-down-down-down."

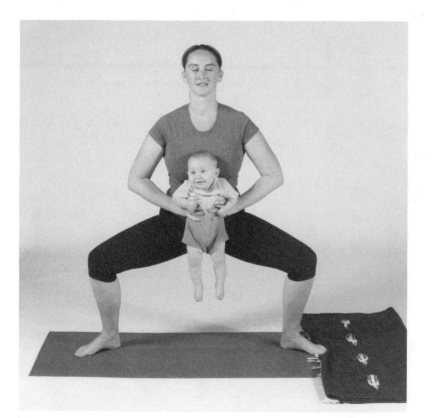

Where's Baby: In your arms, facing whichever way works best for you today

To begin: Stand with your feet a little more than hip width apart. Hold your baby toward you or facing out, whichever feels best today. Inhale. As you exhale, bend your knees, coming down halfway into a squat. As you inhale, squeeze your thighs and buttocks and use your abs as you lift up to a standing position.

Body check: Check your posture. Let your shoulders relax.

Baby check: Does Baby like it?

Repetitions: Five times

Bring one knee down and then the other. Stretch your legs in front of you and bring your baby onto your thighs or against your chest.

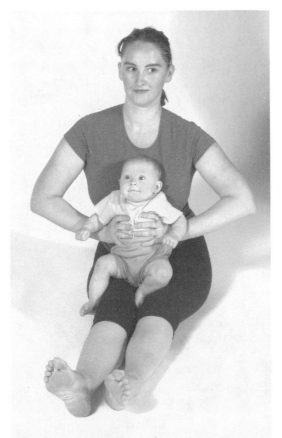

Going Visiting

This movement strengthens your abdominal muscles and tones your buttocks.

Where's Baby: Hold your baby on your lap, facing your chest, until she's two months old. Then she can face out.

To begin: Sit on the floor with your legs extended in front. Use your abs to bring your belly button back toward the spine to support your lower back, and squeeze your buttocks. Breathe comfortably as you "walk" forward in your seated position; bring your right foot forward and then your left, creating a forward motion. Be careful that your baby's legs don't fall between your thighs; if this is happening, hold her under the buttocks. Keep breathing. Keep your chest open and your back tall. Now reverse direction to go backward.

If you are doing this without your baby, use your arms to help with the back-and-forth motion.

Body check: Use your abdominal muscles and squeeze your buttocks together. Lift up through your pelvic floor, keeping your chest open and bringing your shoulder blades on top of your ribs.

Baby check: Make sure Baby is having fun. I like to sing the "Ants Go Marching" song while I go visiting!

Repetitions: Ten steps forward, ten steps backward

Lie down with your baby against your thighs.

Pelvic Tilts

Pelvic tilts strengthen muscles in your lower back, buttocks and abdomen and tone muscles to contribute to healthy circulation.

Where's Baby: Against your thighs. Support her with one or both hands. Babies get a fun little ride as you bring your pelvis up and down!

To begin: Lie down and bend your knees, keeping the soles of your feet on the floor. As you inhale, tilt your pelvis upward. Exhale slowly and bring the pelvis back down and gently contract the abdominal muscles.

Body check: You will feel a gentle massage in your lower back as you bring your pelvis down to the floor.

Repetitions: Do at least three, but you'll probably want to do more because they feel so good.

Now we're going to focus on the abdomen.

Abdominal Work III

While doing abdominal exercises, do the movements slowly, focusing on your abs so you don't use your neck muscles or hip flexors to help you. As you do this version—the crunch—visualize your ribs moving toward the pelvis.

Where's Baby: On a blanket in front of you or against your thighs

To begin: Lie on your back, with your knees bent, soles of the feet on the floor. Put your hands under your head. Exhale and contract your abdominal muscles as you lift your head and shoulders off the floor. Make sure to keep your elbows open out to the side and look up to the ceiling. Inhale, slowly lower your back down to the floor, keeping your abdominals engaged.

Body check: It is important to focus on using your abs to do these movements.

Repetitions: Begin with five and work up to fifteen to twenty.

Abdominal Side-to-Sides

This movement works the muscles on either side of your abdominal recti.

Where's Baby: On a blanket in front of you

To begin: Lie on your back, with your knees bent toward your chest, your feet off the floor and your hands behind your head. Exhale and bring your right elbow across to your bent left knee. Stretch your right leg straight out. Make sure the right shoulder comes off the floor and the left shoulder and upper arm stay on the floor. Inhale, bringing both knees to center. Exhale, bringing your left elbow across to your bent right knee, left leg extended straight. Make sure the left shoulder comes off the floor and the right shoulder and upper arm stay on the floor. Inhale, bringing both knees to center. Repeat.

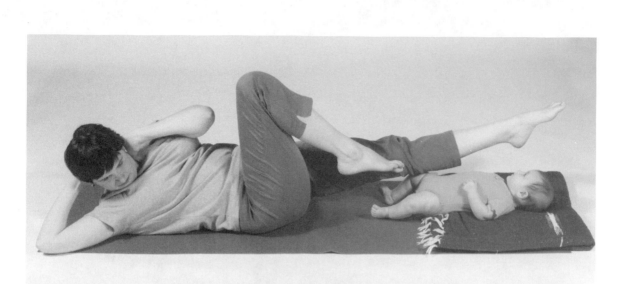

Body check: When you move your right elbow toward your left knee, make sure your left elbow comes to the floor and vice versa.

Repetitions: Five to each side, working up to ten and then fifteen on each side. To finish, bring both knees in to chest, roll side to side and relax.

Stay lying down.

Lift-Ups

This exercise strengthens arms and pectoral muscles, but you'll have to wait to start this until your baby is about twelve weeks old and can hold up his head on his own.

Where's Baby: Hold your baby in your arms.

To begin: Lie on your back, knees bent, with your baby facing you against your chest. Hold your baby around his ribs and tummy. Lift him up over you, say hi and smile, then slowly bring him back down to your chest.

Body check: Contract your abdominals gently so you protect the lower back.

Baby check: Make sure your baby can support his own head.

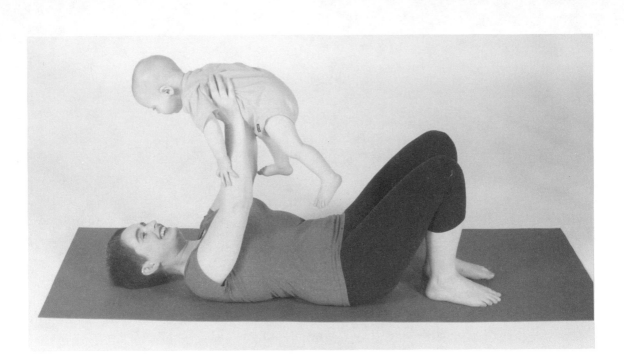

Repetitions: Three times

Bring your baby to your chest and open your knees on either side of your baby.

Knee-to-Chest Rockers

Do a few rocks side to side and then a few rocks forward and back.

Move into the final relaxation pose.

Supported Reclining Pose

This very calming position opens up the chest and helps respiration. Hold as long as you want.

Where's Baby: On a blanket beside you or resting on your belly or chest

Props: Cushion, pillow or blanket

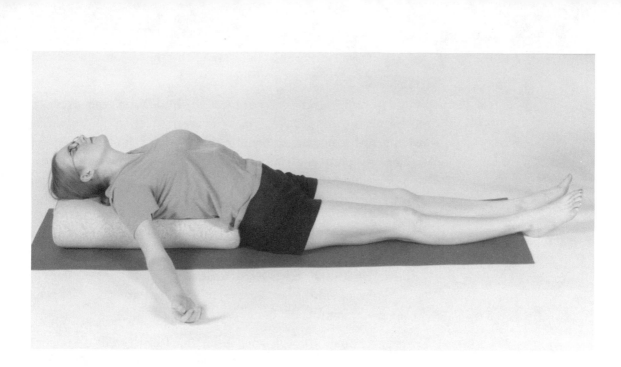

To begin: Lie down on your back on the floor or a bed. Place a cushion between the floor and your back, under your chest area and parallel to your spine. Position your head and chest slightly higher than your abdomen, pelvis and legs. Place two rolled-up blankets under your knees. Let your arms extend away from you, palms facing the sky.

Body check: Make any adjustments to your position so that you are comfortable.

❧ ROUTINE 4 (APPROXIMATELY 50 MINUTES) ❧

Begin in a seated position (cross-legged if it is comfortable for you).

Three-Part Breath (Deergha Swaasam)

This breathing practice calms the body and provides energy and vitality by transporting extra oxygen into the lungs. Deergha

Six to Twelve Weeks

Swaasam also helps turn your awareness to the abdominal muscles as you concentrate on breathing in and out.

This type of breathing can be practiced all the time, whenever you feel a need to center yourself. Whenever I feel anxious or overwhelmed, I remember to breathe this way and I immediately feel better. It is particularly nice to practice this breathing while feeding or holding your baby. The baby picks up on the calmness and positive feeling. Start with ten breaths.

Where's Baby: Held against your chest

To begin: This breathing practice is divided into three parts to best fill the lungs completely. (It will enable you to take seven times as much oxygen into your lungs.) It is easiest to learn Deergha Swaasam by starting out comfortably seated.

Part one: Inhale through your nose, and feel as well as visualize your belly and lower back getting bigger, expanding outward. It is almost as if you are releasing your abdomen up.

Part two: Exhale and feel your belly button move back toward your spine, your abdomen contracting in.

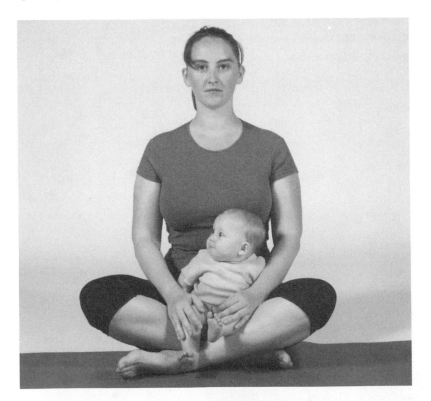

Yoga Mom,
Buddha Baby

Part three: Inhale again, feeling your belly, lower back, rib cage and middle of your back expand. As air continues to enter your lungs, also expand your upper chest; you will feel your collarbone rise. Exhale, feeling your rib cage and belly button coming back in toward your spine.

Forward Neck Release

Do this three times.

Foot Stretch

Make sure to stretch your feet completely.

Come onto your hands and knees.

Wag the Tail

Do this movement three times to each side.

Stay on your hands and knees.

Cat and Cow

Do this flowing movement five times.

Stay on your hands and knees.

Thread the Needle

This is a great stretch for achy upper backs, as it opens up the rib cage, works the waist and stretches the arms, shoulders and back. New moms really like this one for intercostal muscles (the muscles between the ribs).

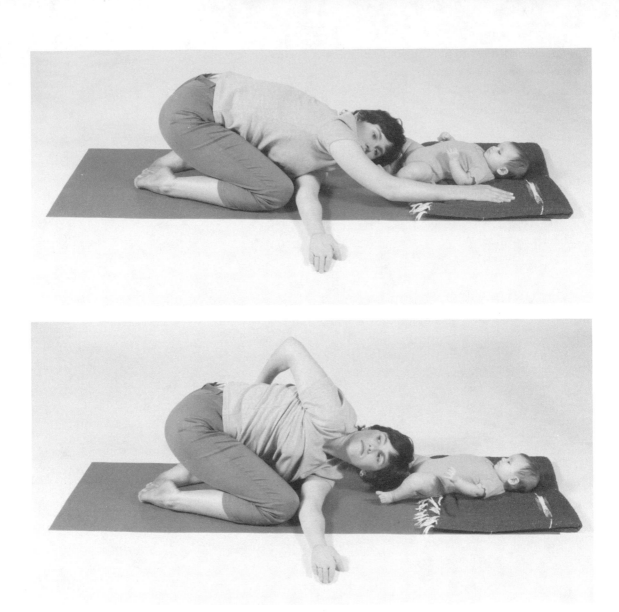

Where's Baby: Close to Mom

To begin: On your hands and knees in the all-fours position, inhale and exhale. Thread your right arm underneath your left arm, bringing your right ear down to the floor. Resting on your right arm and shoulder, raise your left arm toward the ceiling and then wrap it around your back (or leave it on the floor if that's more comfortable). Hold this position for five breaths. Inhale and come back to center. Repeat on your other side, threading your left arm under your right.

Yoga Mom,
Buddha Baby

166

Body check: Make sure the stretch feels gentle throughout.

Repetitions: Do once on each side.

From your hands and knees, sit back.

Child's Pose

Hold as long as you'd like. This is a good position in which to practice your kegels.

Downward Dog

Hold this pose for three breaths.

Stand up slowly by opening your feet a little wider, bending your knees and walking your hands toward your knees to come into a forward standing bend, like a Raggedy Ann doll. Slowly come up by tucking your chin into your chest and rolling up, vertebra by vertebra. Let your head be heavy and then lift up.

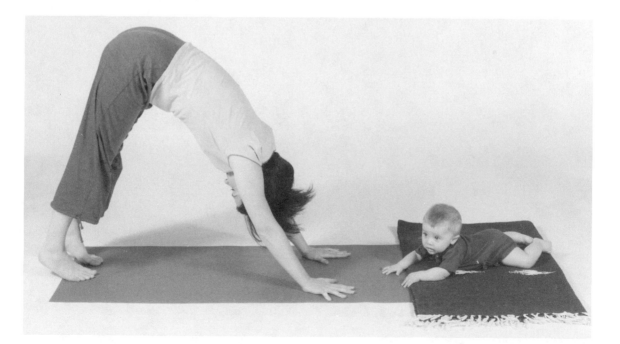

Triangle

One of my favorite poses, triangle strengthens the legs and buttocks, increases flexibility in the spine, stretches side muscles and opens your rib cage, hips and chest.

Where's Baby: On a blanket in front of you

To begin: Stand with your feet a comfortable distance apart (about the length of one leg). Your feet, hips and chest are facing forward; you're standing tall and using your abdominal muscles. Turn your right foot in on a slight angle, then turn your left

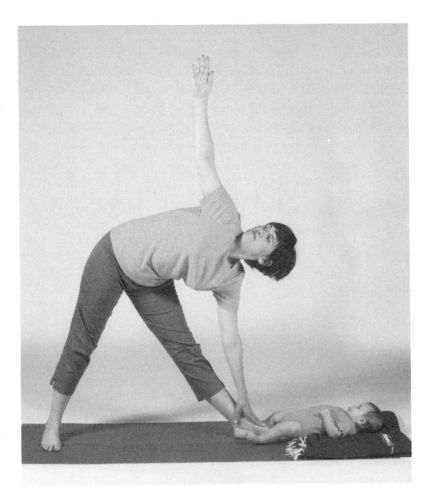

foot to the side. Lift your arms up parallel to the floor and even with your shoulders. Inhale, exhale and stretch to the left side. Inhale, raising your right arm. Exhale and reach your left arm down your left leg. (Advanced yogimamas can bend their left knee, bringing their left elbow to the knee. Cross your right arm behind your back; your left arm goes underneath your left leg to grasp your right hand.) Hold for three breaths. Inhale your body back to center. Switch your foot position and repeat to the right side.

Body check: Feel a good stretch to your side muscles; it does not matter how far down the leg you come.

Repetitions: Hold for three breaths on each side.

Come back to the floor by going into a squat or bringing one knee down and then the other. Turn onto your belly.

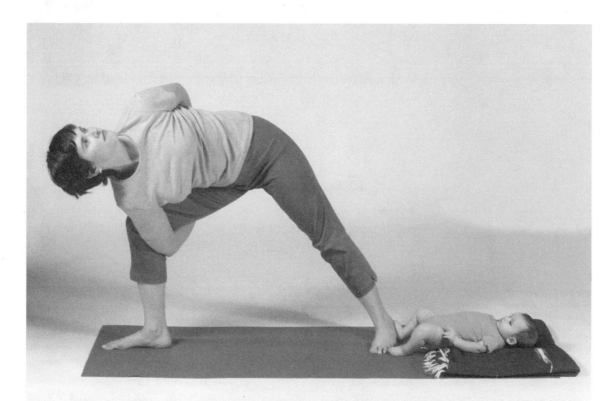

Cobra

Hold for three breaths.

Stay on your belly.

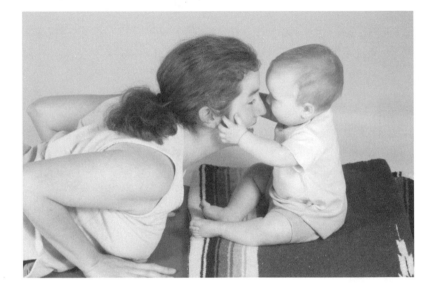

Open Chest Stretch

This terrific stretch releases tension from the chest. It also keeps the spine flexible, works the abdominal muscles and trims the waist. Eastern medical practitioners believe that by stretching the spine, you squeeze out toxins and stimulate the kidneys, spleen and adrenal glands.

Where's Baby: On a blanket in front of you

To begin: Lying on your belly, come onto your forearms, with your elbows below your shoulders. Stretch out your right arm. Inhale and lift your right arm up. Allow the right knee to bend as you bring your arm up and over behind you. You are gazing back toward your open right palm. Breathe easily; hold for three breaths. Inhale and lift your arm up; exhale and bring it back down. Repeat on the other side.

Body check: Stay on your forearms and lift up and out with the arm you are raising. Do not collapse your shoulders.

Repetitions: Do once on each side.

Come onto your back.

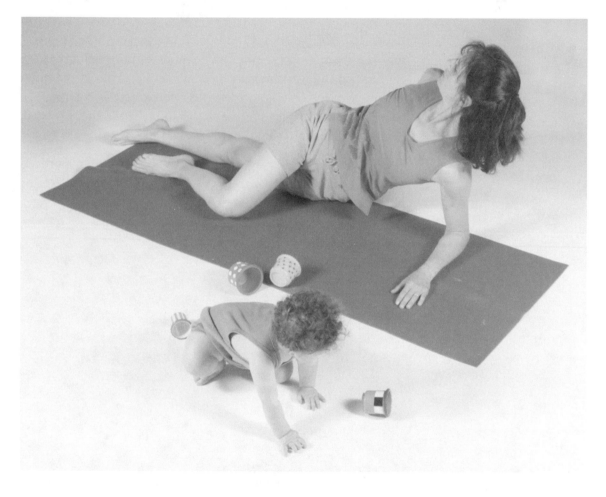

The Bridge

Hold this as long as you like.

Come up to a seated position. Remember to maintain proper posture.

Half Forward Bend
(Janusirasana)

This posture stretches and strengthens the back and hamstrings.

Where's Baby: On a blanket in front of you or in your arms

To begin: Sit with both legs straight out in front of you. Bend your right knee and bring it to the floor, placing your right sole against the left inner thigh. Inhale and reach the arms overhead, lifting from the base of the spine. Exhale; hinge from the hips. Keep lengthening through the spine as you bring your head and chest toward your leg. Take hold of the leg wherever it is comfortable. Let your shoulders relax and surrender into the posture. Use your breath to release into the stretch. Hold for five breaths.

To come out of the posture, stretch both arms out over your feet. Inhale, lifting and reaching up with your arms. Exhale, lowering the arms. Repeat on the other side.

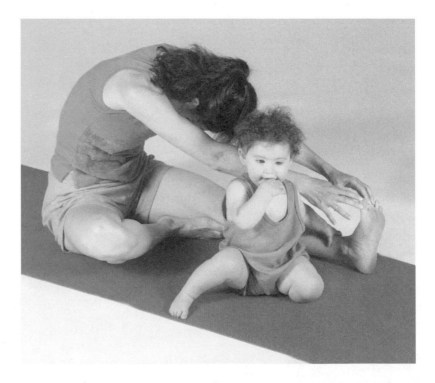

Body check: Keep both buttocks on the floor. You might like to place a blanket under the sits bones. Face the knees and toes of your extended leg up toward the ceiling.

Repetitions: Once on each side, holding for five breaths

Come back down to a lying position.

Knees-to-Chest Rocker

Rock back and forth and side to side several times.

Roll up to a seated position.

Half Spinal Twist
(Ardha Matsyendrasana)

Twist to each side for three breaths.

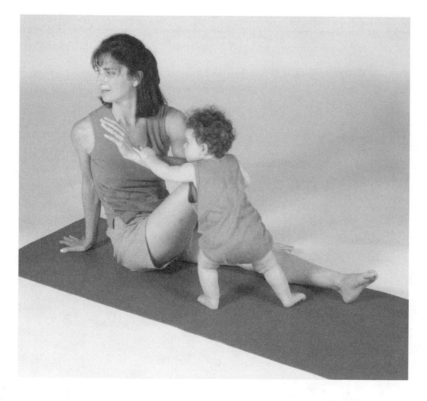

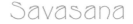

Savasana

Relax in this position as long as you like.

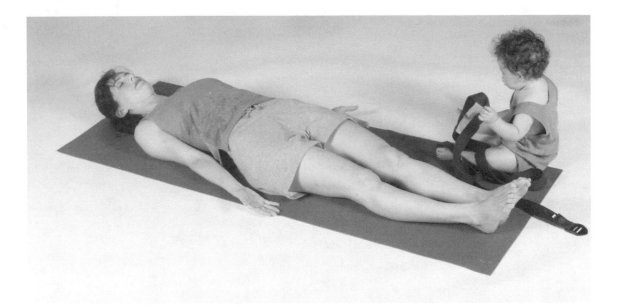

Baby Massage

Massaging a healthy baby helps with mental and physical development and disease preven-
tion. My colleague Durga O'Sullivan, a licensed massage therapist and yoga instructor, shared with
me the techniques she uses to teach mothers how to give wonderful massages to their babies. We
have offered the basics; you may want to get a book devoted to infant massage to learn more
about this special way to relax your baby and to bond with her.

Medical caution: Do not massage a baby if she is sick or has a fever.

It's important when you massage your baby that you give her your whole focus. It's also important to be gentle in your movements, and to always watch your baby to make sure she is enjoying the massage motions.

Before you begin, make sure the environment is right for your baby. Consider the temperature, lighting and surrounding sounds. Is the room warm enough? It's best for your baby to be naked during massage, but if the room is not warm, dress her in smooth, simple clothes. Also make sure there aren't any drafts. The lighting should be soft; your baby won't want to stare up at a bright light. And the room should be quiet, without the TV blaring or the window open if there is a lot of traffic noise.

Good times for giving your baby a massage are around nap time, before or after a bath or before she goes to bed. Do not give a massage after your baby has just eaten. If your baby pulls away from your strokes or is cranky, stop the massage and try again later or another day.

Durga always reminds the moms she works with to convey confidence when giving their baby a massage. Don't worry that you are not an "expert masseuse"—as a mother, anytime you touch your baby you are the expert. She suggests that the touch match the energy of your baby; some babies like a stronger touch and stroke pressure, others a more delicate one, so watch your baby's reaction. Always massage gently, keeping both hands on your baby as much as possible; this will ground the energy and make your baby feel safe and comfortable. And you will also want to connect with your baby, so make eye contact and hold him.

Massage strokes should be done with an open palm. Do not knead or use fingertips; babies like smooth strokes. Let your palms and fingers mold with your baby to melt and be one with his body. Use smooth, evenly energized strokes, with the pressure matched to your baby's preference.

Massage oil helps create smooth, gliding strokes while also moisturizing baby's skin. If you decide to use an oil:

- always apply a little bit to your baby's skin prior to using it if you are worried about an allergy
- always apply the oil to your palms and not directly onto your baby's skin
- make sure the oil is warm by rubbing your palms together or putting the jar of oil in warm water

I recommend using an unscented natural oil; almond and sesame oil are particularly nice, and coconut oil is a fun treat in the summer.

BASIC BABY MASSAGE

Where's Baby: Always position your baby on her back, looking up. Make sure she is in a warm, draft-free space. Where you put your baby will depend on his size. You can put your baby on a soft towel or baby blanket on the floor in front of you. You can also put him on you by sitting with both legs out and your baby lying across you or on your legs with him positioned lap to feet. Whatever position you choose, make sure you are comfortable; leaning against pillows on a bed works well.

Beginning the Massage Place both warm, open palms on baby's belly to make initial contact. As a nice opening chant you can try: "Open your heart and lungs to me/Open your spirit and soul to me." Then slowly spread your hands away from each other, away from the center of the belly. Use gentle strokes to familiarize your baby with the contact and to ground both of you.

Chest Bring both hands to the top of your baby's chest, in the middle over the breastbone. Gently move both hands down and toward either side, using slow, even strokes. Stop at the edge of his chest and bring your hands back to the top and center. Repeat strokes up to eight times.

Shoulder to Hip Position both hands on the left shoulder. Keep one hand gently on the shoulder and with the other stroke down toward the right hip. Lift your hand and bring it back to the shoulder. Repeat three times. Now repeat strokes from the right shoulder to the left hip.

Belly Place both hands just above the groin. Using both hands, stroke up from the groin, around the navel and back down. Make three to six rotations.

Arms and Hands *Milking:* Hold the shoulder with one hand. Wrap your other palm across your baby's arm and stroke down to the wrist. Repeat three times.

Wringing: Wrap both hands around your baby's arm. Stroke as though you are (gently!) wringing out a towel by moving your hands in opposite directions. Start at the shoulder and go down to the wrist. Repeat once.

Finish the arm massage by gently massaging his palms with your thumb pads (not nails). Push your thumbs lightly against his palm and move your thumbs from the center out. Repeat in all directions as if drawing sun rays from the center of his palm.

Repeat with the other arm.

Legs and Feet *Milking:* Hold the hip with one hand. Wrap your other palm across your baby's leg and stroke down to the ankle. Repeat three times.

Wringing: Wrap both hands around your baby's leg. Stroke as though you are (gently!) wringing out a towel by moving your hands in opposite directions. Start at the hip and go down to the ankle. Repeat once.

Complete the leg massage by gently massaging the soles of his feet with your thumb pads (not nails). Push your thumbs gently against his sole and move your thumbs from the center out. Repeat in all directions.

Repeat with the other leg.

Back Bring both hands under your baby, one hand on top of the other, palms facing up against his spine. Open your fingers to form a V so that as you stroke down his spine, your fingers are spread to create space for the vertebrae. Using steady pressure, stroke down his spine as if you were "ironing" his back, putting the pressure on either side of the vertebrae. As with all strokes, use even, gentle pressure. Repeat up to four times.

Face Rest the pads of your fingers on the bridge of his nose and gently stroke up to the forehead. Trace the eyes and around the nose, cheekbones and chin with gentle strokes, using your finger pads. You can also make little circles on his forehead. Be creative. A massage of the face should be calming to your baby. If your baby is not happy, do not continue.

Finishing the Massage Place the center of your palm on top of his head and your other palm on top and just below his navel. Keep your hands in place, using very light pressure. Slowly leave his body, bringing your hands directly up. Your baby will think you are still there—and your energy is!

Massaging Older Babies It is generally easier to massage babies before they start crawling (six months). After six months, you may find it easier to massage parts of the body rather than give a full massage.

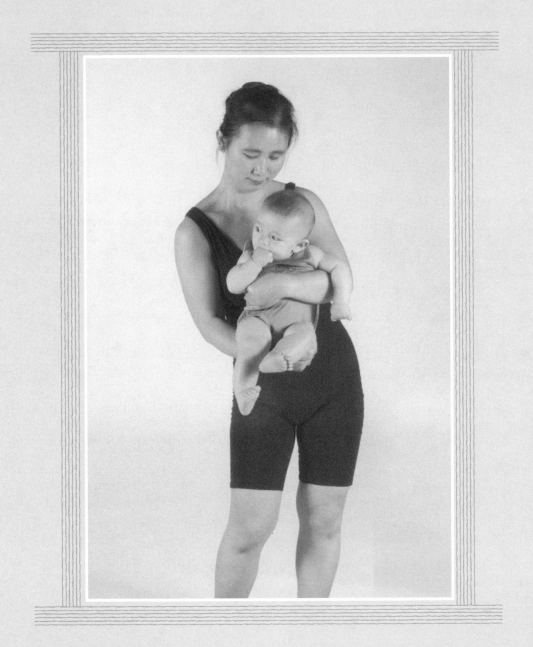

Ten

Three Months to One Year

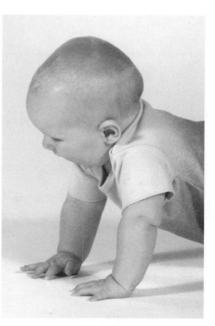

Soon your baby will begin to do her own cobra: watch her push down on her palms, raising her head and pushing up to see even more. The world becomes bigger to her as she learns to lift her head and becomes more mobile. This means even more interaction and fun as you practice your yoga with your baby.

This period also marks more changes in motherhood and your body. You are not only looking after and responsible for this amazing being, but you are also looking after your changing self. There will be days when you feel you've really gotten it together and other days when you feel you can't cope. Don't be hard on yourself. As a friend of mine observes, "Motherhood is right up there next to sainthood." Please enjoy this time. It's amazing to me that when my children were babies, sometimes five minutes felt like five hours, yet now when I look at them I sometimes

Three Months to
One Year

179

wonder where all the time has gone. So my advice as a mother is to breathe and take things a moment at a time, because "the days are long, the years go fast."

Also at this stage, moms usually start asking me about getting their shape back and taking off the extra pounds. We are all different, so how your body changes will depend on who you are. Give yourself at least a year; do yoga and love your body. Look at all it is doing!

❧ ROUTINE 1 (APPROXIMATELY 20 MINUTES) ❧

Begin in a seated position (cross-legged if it is comfortable for you).

Half Neck Rolls

I hope you've been using these to relieve neck and shoulder tension throughout the day. Relax your shoulders during this movement. If an area feels achy or tight, breathe into that spot to let go of tension. As you inhale, visualize bringing oxygen to the tight area; as you exhale, breathe out the tension. Notice if one side feels tighter than the other; what do you do differently on that side of the body? If you hear cracks or pops, it's just tension being released from the joints.

As you do the neck rolls, you may find that you want to sigh or moan or groan. Please do! This helps relieve tension and makes your jaw and facial muscles relax. Do at least two to each side.

Shoulder Rolls

Shoulder rolls open up the chest and upper back and relieve tension in the shoulders. This posture helps moms who hold their baby in a front carrier, especially as your baby gets heavier. Do these whenever you need to! Start with at least three circles in each direction. You may like doing the shoulder roll in one direction more than you do the other. Check both out and see which you prefer.

Come onto your hands and knees.

Child's Pose

Child's pose provides a great stretch for the spine, in addition to relaxing your entire body and mind.

Where's Baby: Lying in front of you. When you come down, wiggle your head to tickle your baby with your hair or give your baby a "raspberry" on her belly.

To begin: From your hands and knees, open your knees a little wider, bringing your toes together and your heels apart. Move your buttocks back to rest between your heels, bringing your forehead down toward the floor. Breathe and relax. You can either keep your arms crossed under your forehead, stretched straight above your head or stretched out back along your body—whichever you find most comfortable. Rest in child's pose as long as you need to feel the tension dissolve from your body and your mind quieting. Concentrate on slow, rhythmic breathing.

Body check: Be aware of being comfortable; use blankets or pillows under your knees or chest if desired.

Repetitions: Once, twice or as many times as you need throughout the day. This is a great posture on its own. It's a great back stretch and also a great position in which to do kegels.

Come back up onto your hands and knees.

Downward Dog

This is a terrific stretching movement for the back and hamstrings. It also strengthens the upper body and tones your abdominals.

Where's Baby: Lying in front of you

To begin: Begin on your hands and knees. Make sure there is space between your fingers. Curl your toes underneath. Inhale, and as you exhale, push up, moving your buttocks up toward the ceiling in an inverted V. Bring your belly button toward the spine and press your heels down toward the floor. Open up between your shoulder blades, let your head relax and look at your knees.

Time: Stay in this position for at least three breaths or as long as is comfortable.

Walk the dog variation: While in downward dog, raise your left heel, bending the left knee. Now bring the right heel down toward the floor and hold for ten seconds. Raise your right heel and bring your left heel to the floor, holding for ten seconds. Finish by bringing both heels back down toward the floor.

Body check: Be aware of the feet and legs; they should be close together. Let the shoulders relax. Make sure not to lock your elbows (hyperextension weakens the ligaments).

Repetitions: Do once, holding for three breaths.

Come down onto your belly.

Cobra

This pose tones and strengthens the upper and lower back and abdominal muscles. It also massages internal organs and opens up the thyroid gland.

Where's Baby: In front of you

To begin: Lying on your belly, bring your palms underneath your shoulders. Bring your forehead to the floor, making sure your legs and feet are also on the floor. As you inhale, lengthen from the base of your spine and reach out from the crown of the head. Your nose and chin will brush the mat. Using your palms for gentle sup-

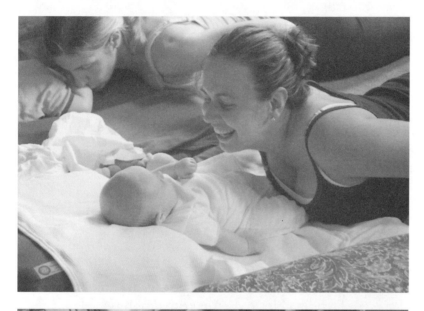

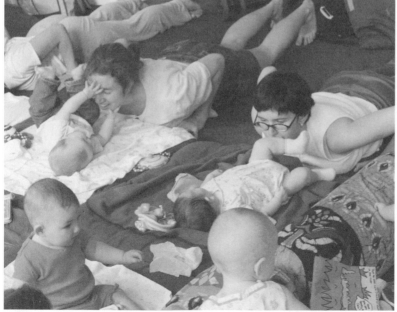

port, lift your upper body forward and up, opening up through the chest. Keep your shoulders relaxed and your elbows slightly bent alongside the body. Lift your belly up to the spine using your abs, but keep your pelvis on the floor. Take three gentle breaths. Slowly lower back down, vertebra by vertebra, allowing your chin to touch the mat first, and then your forehead. Turn your head to the side. Bring your arms alongside your body and relax. You can also relax into child's pose.

From here you can do push-ups over your baby, coming down to give her kisses or nookies on her belly.

Body check: Keep your pelvis on the floor.

Repetitions: Do once, taking three breaths.

Roll over onto your back.

Pelvic Tilts

Pelvic tilts strengthen muscles in your lower back, buttocks and abdomen and tone muscles to contribute to healthy circulation.

Where's Baby: Against your thighs. Support her with one or both hands. Babies get a fun little ride as you bring your pelvis up and down!

To begin: Lie down and bend your knees, keeping the soles of your feet on the floor. As you inhale, tilt your pelvis upward. Exhale slowly, bring the pelvis down, and gently contract the abdominal muscles.

Body check: You will feel a gentle massage in your lower back as you bring your pelvis down to the floor.

Repetitions: Begin with three. These feel great, so do more if you like.

Sit up.

Full Forward Bend
(Paschimottanasana)

This pose stretches back and leg muscles and tones abdominal organs.

Where's Baby: On a blanket in front of you or in your arms

To begin: Sit with your legs stretched out in front of you. Inhale and lift your arms overhead. As you exhale, hinge from your hips, stretching your arms and body out over your extended legs. Take hold of your legs wherever is most comfortable. Let your head, neck and shoulders relax. Breathe and surrender into the pose. Hold for five breaths.

If you are doing this posture while holding your baby she will be facing you. Inhale, lengthening the spine. As you exhale, hinge forward at the hips. Bring your baby onto your legs as you come

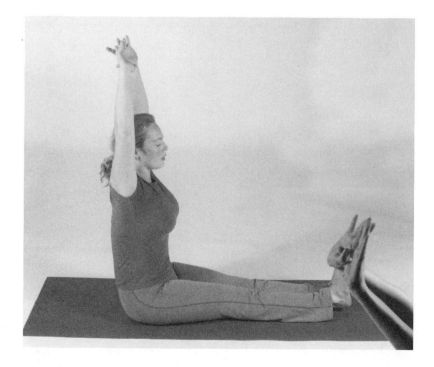

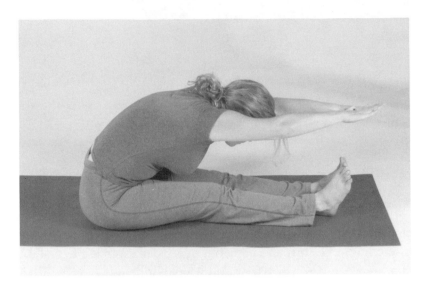

forward. Breathe and surrender into the pose for five breaths. Give kisses to your baby.

To come out of the forward bend, inhale and stretch out and up and raise yourself back to a seated position. Lift your baby up with you. Exhale and lower your arms.

To lie down for shoulder stand, you can come from sitting to slowly lying all the way down, using your abdominals.

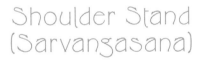

Shoulder Stand (Sarvangasana)

This inverted posture lets the blood from the lower body move in the opposite direction to the upper body and is good for circulation. It also tones the buttocks, lengthens the spine and improves balance. In addition, this upside-down pose tones the thyroid, helps with varicose veins and is good for the heart, lungs and nervous system.

Medical cautions: Do not do shoulder stands if you are menstruating or have neck or eye problems.

Where's Baby: On a blanket beside you

To begin: Tuck in your shirt and lift any long hair away from your neck. Lie down with your legs together and your arms alongside your body. You may want to put a blanket under your shoulders for cushioning. Press your palms into the floor and raise your legs—while keeping them straight—to a ninety-degree angle. If your lower back is achy, bend your knees and then bring your legs to a ninety-degree angle. With your legs pointing to the sky, push down through your palms and swing your legs over your head so that they are now parallel to the floor. Place your palms on the middle of your back for support. Raise your legs up to a vertical position. Bring your chest toward your chin. (You may want to lean your legs against the wall

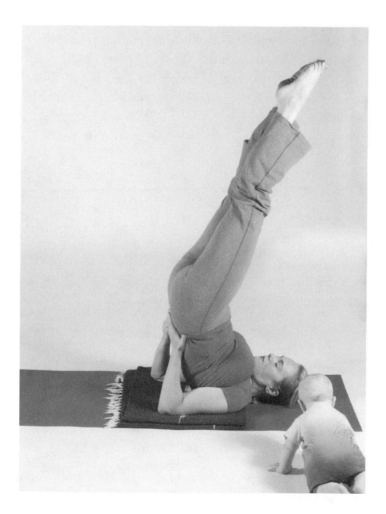

for added support.) Keep your feet together, with your toes slightly pointed toward the sky. Relax your face and your breathing. Keep your neck still. Hold your shoulder stand for two minutes. If you feel any discomfort, come out of the pose.

Coming out of the pose: Slowly lower your legs over your head until they are parallel with the floor. Continue to use your hands for support against your back. With your legs parallel to the floor, slowly lower your back to the floor vertebra by vertebra. Keeping your knees straight, slowly lower your legs to the floor as well. You can also bend your knees and bring the soles of the feet to the floor (if there is lower-back achiness.) Do not lift your head or back up; contract your abdominals as you lower your legs down. Rest. If you are feeling strain in your lower back, bring your knees to your chest.

Body check: When coming into shoulder stand, if your lower back is achy, bend your knees with the soles of the feet on the floor. For extra cushioning, place your shoulders on the edge of a blanket and let your head and neck come off the blanket. You will get the most benefit if your legs stay up, but if you want you can do scissors—bringing one leg back at a time—or open your legs in a V.

The Plow

This advanced posture feels good, providing an intense stretch in the neck and lower back. But go into it slowly!

Medical cautions: Skip this if you are experiencing any neck or other medical problems. Do not do the plow if you are menstruating or have neck or eye problems.

Where's Baby: On a blanket beside you

To begin: From shoulder stand, lower your legs down toward the floor behind your head. Keep your legs straight. Bend your knees around your ears and wrap your arms around your knees.

To come out: Straighten your legs and come back into shoulder stand. Now come down from shoulder stand, bending your knees and slowly bringing your legs down.

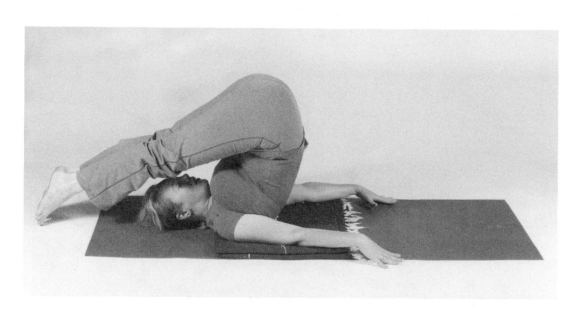

Body check: Use your abdominals to lower your legs. Breathe and relax.

Repetitions: Do once, holding for five breaths.

Fish Pose (Matsyaasana)

This is a complementary pose to shoulder stand, so always do this pose after shoulder stand or plow. This pose stretches the thyroid gland in the opposite direction from shoulder stand. This is also a great chest opener.

Where's Baby: On a blanket beside you

To begin: Lie on your back with your legs together. Take hold of the sides of your thighs with your hands. With your weight on your elbows and forearms, start opening up your belly, ribs and chest and bring the crown of your head down toward the floor. There will be a pronounced arch in your back. Your weight is balanced between your buttocks and elbows and the top of your head. Feel your chest opening up. Take three nice deep breaths. The lungs are really open in this pose.

To come out of fish pose, push down on your elbows. Bring your head up, look at your feet and slowly roll down to the floor, verte-

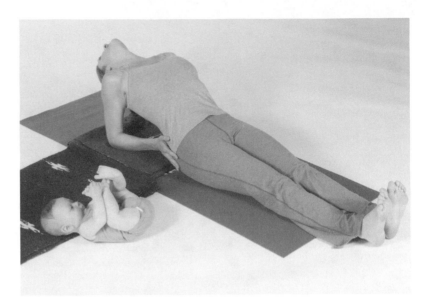

bra by vertebra. Hug your knees to your chest and roll your head from side to side.

Body check: Distribute your weight so that there is no strain on your neck. For a restorative variation, place a cushion under your back, letting your head and neck come off the cushion.

Repetitions: Do once, holding for at least three breaths.

Come up to a sitting position.

Half Spinal Twist (Ardha Matsyendrasana)

This pose does much more than tone the abdominal area—it also stretches the back and side muscles, helps with digestive problems, keeps the spine flexible, squeezes toxins out of the spine as if one is "wringing a washcloth", and massages internal organs.

Where's Baby: Close to you or sitting with you

To begin: In a seated position, stretch your legs out in front of you. Keep your left leg straight as you cross your right foot over your left knee. Keep sitting up tall. Bring your right hand behind your spine. Bring your left arm around to the outside of your right knee. Twist and look over your right shoulder. Breathe comfortably, using your breath to help you stretch. Inhale and sit up tall; exhale and let the breath move you a little farther into the twist. Stay there, holding for three breaths.

To come out of this pose, inhale and bring your head back to center. Exhale and release your arms. Inhale, exhale and look over your left shoulder. Return to center. Repeat on the other side.

Body check: Keep both buttocks on the floor. Check your posture; make sure you have a tall back.

Repetitions: Do once on each side.

Yoga Mudra

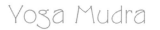

This position seals in the positive energy that you've created in your body from the postures you've completed.

Where's Baby: On a blanket in front of you

To begin: Sit in a comfortable position with your legs crossed. Bring your hands behind your back. Take hold of your right wrist with your left hand. Inhale, lengthen through the spine. As you exhale, hinge forward from the hips, bringing your forehead toward the floor. Breathe and bring your awareness inward. Relax

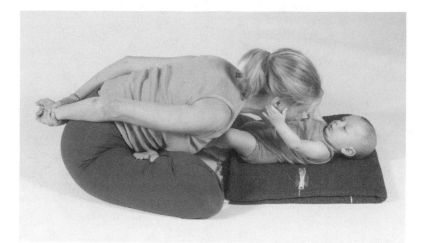

your head, neck and shoulders. Surrender. Let your tension go. Hold for five breaths.

To come out of yoga mudra, reach out with the crown of your head as you inhale and come up. Return your hands to your knees, palms upward in receiving position.

Body check: Feel the stretch in your back as you bring your forehead to the floor, and then let go.

Repetitions: Do once, holding for five breaths.

Lie down for the final relaxation pose.

Supported Bound Angle (Supta Baddha Konasana)

This is a terrific position for quick rejuvenation. The pose opens the hip and groin area, encouraging blood flow. It also helps alleviate backaches. It opens up the chest, which is great for moms be-

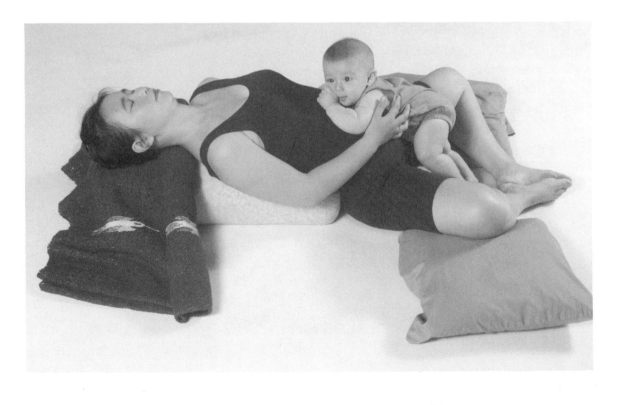

cause you may feel as if your shoulders are really slumped forward. Hold as long as you want.

Medical cautions: Do not do this pose if you have any nerve problems in your neck or spinal disk conditions.

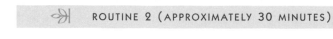

ROUTINE 2 (APPROXIMATELY 30 MINUTES)

Begin in a seated position (cross-legged if it is comfortable for you).

Three-Part Breath (Deergha Swaasam)

This breathing practice calms the body and provides energy and vitality by transporting extra oxygen into the lungs. Deergha

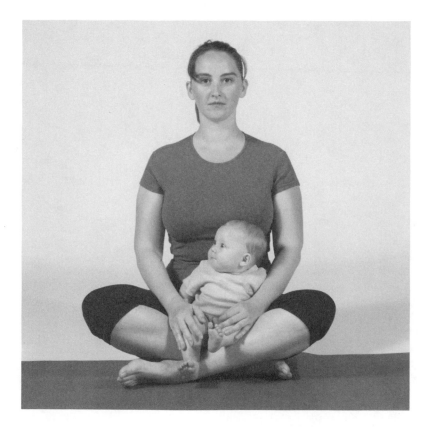

Swaasam also helps turn your awareness to the abdominal muscles as you concentrate on breathing in and out.

This type of breathing can be practiced all the time, whenever you feel a need to center yourself. Whenever I feel anxious or overwhelmed I remember to breathe this way and I immediately feel better. It is particularly nice to practice this breathing while feeding or holding your baby. The baby picks up on the calmness and positive feeling.

Forward Neck Release

This movement releases tension in your neck, shoulders and upper back. It also provides a nice stretch for the vertebrae in the cervical spine.

Do the entire sequence two or three times.

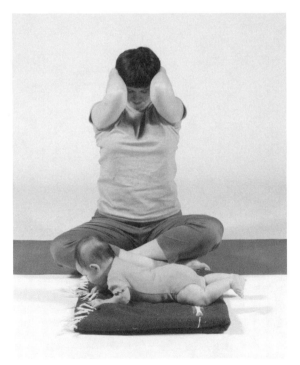 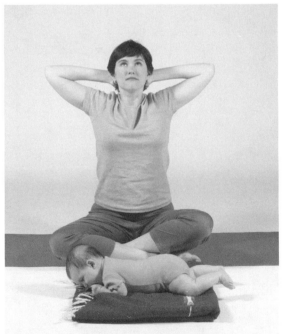

Foot Stretch

This stretch loosens your calf muscles, encourages blood circulation in your lower limbs and minimizes swelling in the feet and ankles.

Where's Baby: Hold your baby or rest her in your lap. As you wiggle your toes, you can wiggle hers, as well as rotate her ankles gently and play games with her toes.

To begin: Give all your toes a nice wiggle. Rotate your ankles gently to the right, making a slow clockwise circle. Now rotate in the other direction. Do five circles in each direction.

Next, flex your feet, stretching your heels away from you as you point your toes toward yourself. Hold for several seconds and release. Do this flex exercise for one minute.

Now stand up and stretch your toes like duck feet, imagining webs between your toes. Lift your toes off the floor and then return them to the floor, two to three times for each foot.

Body check: Make sure your whole body is comfortable. We tend to neglect the feet, so take some time with this stretch.

Pregnancy tends to flatten out feet. In standing poses you can lift your toes off the floor during a stretch; this will create an arch.

Repetitions: Stretch both feet for about one minute per foot. Do foot circles five times in each direction or as often as you desire.

Come onto your hands and knees and sit back.

Child's Pose

Hold this pose for three breaths; it's a good pose during which to practice kegels.

Move back into an all-fours position to push up into downward dog.

Downward Dog

Hold this for at least three breaths.

Stand up slowly by opening your feet a little wider, bending your knees and walking your hands toward your knees to come into a forward standing bend. You'll slowly rise by tucking your chin into your chest and rolling up, vertebra by vertebra, your head coming up last.

Warrior

Warrior pose is another favorite of mine, because doing this pose strengthens my spirit. It also strengthens the thighs, opens the chest, rib cage and back and helps with your sense of balance.

Where's Baby: On a blanket in front of you or in your arms. If you are holding your baby she can face either away from or toward you.

To begin: Stand with your feet together, arms at your sides. Check your posture—think "belly button back toward spine"—and lift the belly button up. Bring your right leg forward about one leg length in front of your left leg. Your right foot should be facing forward; pivot your left foot to a slight angle. Bend your right knee forward, so the right knee is in line over the right ankle. For advanced yogimamas, work to get your right thigh parallel to the floor. Bring your hands into a prayer position, then lift your arms over your head. Feel the lift come from the bottom of the rib cage. Relax your shoulders. If

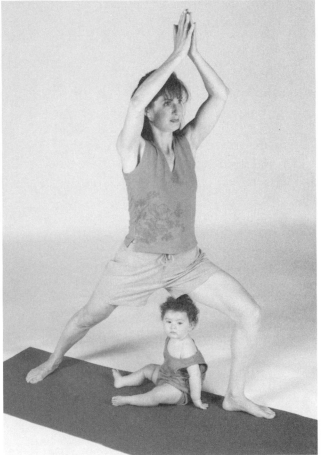

Yoga Mom,
Buddha Baby

196

you're comfortable, bring your gaze gently upward. This is a big stretch—the lower body pushes down into the earth while the upper body lifts up toward the heavens. Hold for five breaths.

To release, bring your arms down into prayer position. Release your arms along your body. Straighten your front leg. Turn both legs and hips to face forward. Step your feet together. Repeat on the other side.

If you are strong enough, you can hold your baby as you do warrior pose, as long as he is able to hold up his head on his own.

Body check: Press the lower body down toward the earth. Lift up the pelvic floor and reach your upper body, lifting from the lowest rib, toward the heavens. Use your abdominals.

Lie down on your back.

Pelvic Tilts

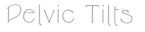

Do three pelvic tilts with your baby on your thighs for a fun little ride.

Stay on your back.

Leg Lifts with Babies (Baby Rides)

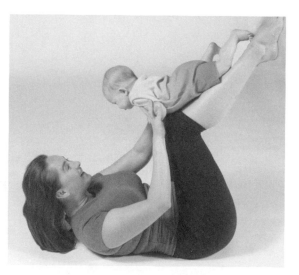

This movement strengthens the abdominal muscles and tones buttocks.

Where's Baby: On Mom's shins, getting little leg lifts as Mom works her abs. I love this movement and still do these with Mikela.

To begin: Lie on your back with your knees toward your chest; your baby is resting on your shins, with you holding her there. Bring your head and neck off the floor. Feel your abdominals engage. Do little leg lifts to move baby up and down.

Body check: If your neck gets sore, bring your head down to the floor and turn it from side to side. Usually if you are focused and engaging your abdominals, your neck won't hurt.

Repetitions: As many as you and your baby want

Put your baby down next to you.

Shoulder Stand

Hold for three minutes.

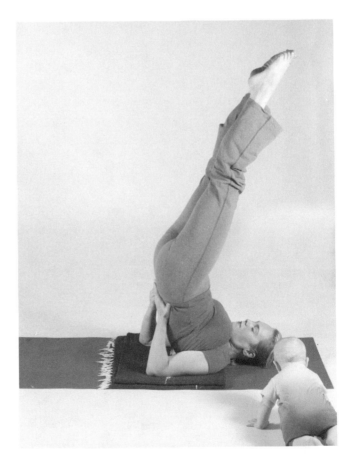

Fish Pose

Hold for three breaths.

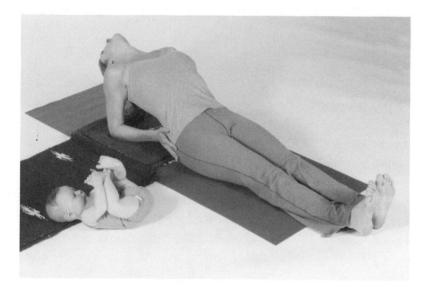

Knees-to-Chest Rocker

This movement massages your lower-back muscles to relieve tightness and tension.

Where's Baby: Lying at your side or resting on your shins. When you rock forward and back, your baby loves the ride.

To begin: Lie on your back, legs and arms straight. Bring your knees up and to your chest and wrap your arms around your legs so you are rolled into a ball. As you feel your lower back opening up, rock gently from side to side, giving your back a massage. Next rock front to back, massaging your spine. Slowly bring your hands away and lower your arms and legs to the floor.

Body check: Enjoy!

Repetitions: Rock as long as it feels good.

Baby Crocodile
Spinal Twist

This posture opens the chest and hips and gently stretches your spine.

Where's Baby: On a blanket in front of you

To begin: Lie on your back with your knees bent to your chest. Extend your arms out to the side, keeping them on the floor perpendicular to your body. Bring both knees together over to the right side of your body and turn your head to the left. Hold this posture as long as you like. Then bring the left knee over to the other side. When your right knee doesn't stay down anymore, bring it over to the left side too. Turn your head to the right. Hold as long as you like. Bring your head and knees back to center, hold, then extend each leg out so that you are lying down with your legs stretched out.

Body check: Make sure both shoulders stay on the floor. You might also place a cushion under your knees if they don't come all the way down to the floor.

Gentle alternative: Lie on your back with your arms around your midsection. Lower the knees from side to side, gently and slowly. Take time to move into the twist.

Repetitions: Once on each side

Move into relaxation.

The yoga for me changes over time; you learn about your baby as they have different growth spurts. Doing yoga postures with her for health benefits is different from putting your child with a baby-sitter and going to a yoga class without her. My mother thinks Stella is relaxed because of yoga.

—JODY AND DAUGHTER STELLA

Savasana

This posture helps bring deep relaxation to your entire body while quieting the mind. It is a good position to do with three-part breath.

Props: Cushion, pillow or blanket

Where's Baby: Next to you

To begin: Lie down on your back with a cushion, pillow or rolled-up blanket tucked under your bent knees. You can also do savasana without any props. Place a small rolled-up blanket under your neck and put a blanket over yourself for warmth, if needed. Breathe fluidly and let your mind and body relax.

Body check: Make any adjustments to your position so that you are comfortable.

Length: As long as you want

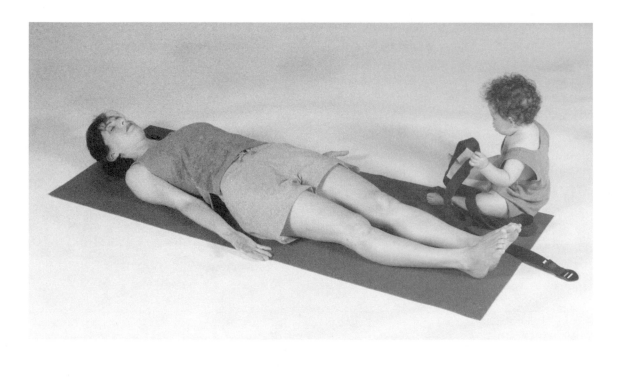

Baby Moves

Here are some more baby moves appropriate to this age group, and you can also keep doing the baby moves introduced in the earlier chapters.

BABY SIT-UPS AND STAND-UPS

Baby sit-ups strengthen your baby's back and neck muscles. You may still need to support your baby's head, although usually by three months, babies hold up their own heads. Then, you can progress to stand-ups, as she moves from lying down to sitting to standing up. How exciting! Have fun!

To begin: Lie your baby on her back. Take hold of her hands and gently, slowly help her come to a sitting position. Then slowly, gently help her roll back down. Be creative; be involved. Encourage her with "Baby going up, up, up Baby going down, down, down." As your baby gets older, she will want to pull up to standing from her sitting position. Encourage her with smiles and a "yay!"

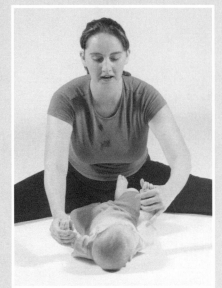

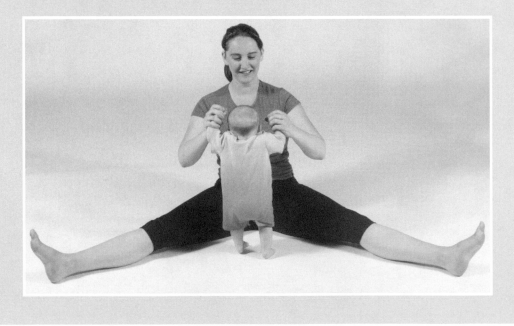

Baby check: Make sure your baby is enjoying this.

Repetitions: Once

BABY INVERSION

This pose is good for circulation; it allows blood and lymphatic fluids to flow from the legs toward the upper body, benefiting the nervous system.

   To begin: Sit with your legs stretched out in front of you and place your baby on your legs, with her head just above your ankles. Bend your knees slowly, thus bringing your baby into a slight inversion. Support her body with your arms. Hold for ten seconds or longer if your baby likes it. Then slowly lower your legs. Let your baby lie down for a few moments, then bring her into a sitting position.

   Repetition: Do once.

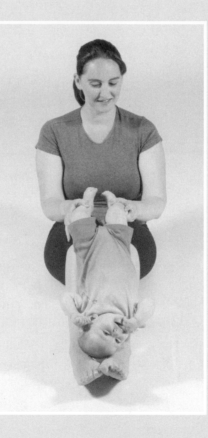

Begin in a seated position (cross-legged if it is comfortable for you).

Half Neck Rolls

With your baby in your lap, do twenty of these.

Shoulder Rolls

Do as many shoulder rolls as you need to relax and open your shoulders.

Put your baby down and come onto your hands and knees.

Wag the Tail

This movement gives a good stretch to the muscles between the ribs.

Where's Baby: Lying in front of you on a blanket

To begin: Come onto your hands and knees. Position your palms under your shoulders and your knees under your hips. Lift your belly button up toward your spine. Contracting your abdominal muscles, inhale. As you exhale, look over your right shoulder as you push out your right hip, bringing your right shoulder and right hip toward each other. Inhale back to center. Move your head from side to side, letting your baby grab your hair. Then repeat on the other side.

Body check: Contract your abdominal muscles as you do this pose.

Repetitions: Three times on each side

Child's Pose

Hold as long as you like; this is a good pose during which to practice your kegels.

Stand up slowly by opening your feet a little wider, bending your knees and walking your hands toward your knees to come into an upright position. Pick up your baby and slowly stand.

Flying Babies

This slow, gentle motion soothes and entertains your baby while building strength in your arms, back and chest.

Where's Baby: Being held by you, facing out

To begin: Part one: Stand with your feet a comfortable distance apart. Hold your baby against your chest (facing outward), with one or both hands under her buttocks. Inhale, exhale and lift your baby to the right as you bring your weight to the right side. Your knees will bend and then straighten when your baby is all the way over to the right. Reverse and "fly" your baby to the left side. This should be a slow, gentle movement.

Body check: Let your shoulders relax. Put on some favorite music and, as always, check your posture, breathe and enjoy.

Baby check: Make sure your baby is enjoying the motion; gauge whether to pick up the pace or slow it down on the basis of her reaction.

Repetitions: A few times on each side

If your baby liked this, then try this second variation:

Part two: Hold your baby in a football hold, with her lying down on your forearm, your palm upward toward her belly and your other hand on her back. Come down into a squat, then lift your baby into a high dive. Lower your baby toward the ground—the low dive. Check your baby's response to know whether to continue, perhaps make smaller dives or stop altogether for today.

Half Squats with Babies

This movement, using your baby as a "weight," works on the arms, thighs and buttocks. As you do this pose, you can say to your baby "Baby goes up-up-up-up-up," then "Baby goes down-d-down-d-down."

Where's Baby: In your arms, facing whichever way works best for you today

To begin: Stand with your feet a little more than hip width apart. Hold your baby toward you or facing out, whichever feels best today; make sure one hand supports your baby's center of gravity

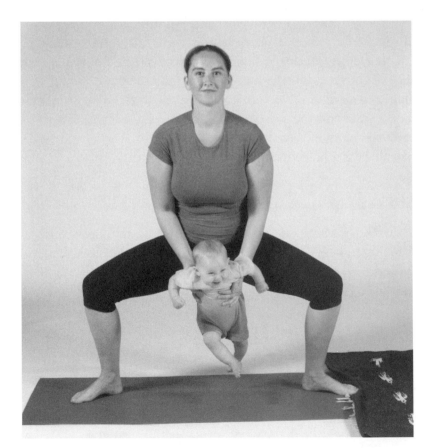

(under her buttocks). Inhale. As you exhale, bend your knees, coming down halfway into a squat. As you inhale, squeeze your thighs and buttocks and use your abs as you lift up to a standing position.

Body check: Check your posture. Let your shoulders relax.

Baby check: Does Baby like it?

Repetitions: Five times

Come down to the floor in a seated position, with your legs stretched out in front of you.

Going Visiting

This movement strengthens your abdominal muscles and tones your buttocks.

Where's Baby: Hold your baby on your lap, facing out.

To begin: Sit on the floor with your legs extended in front of you. Use your abs to bring your belly button back toward the spine to support your lower back. Squeeze your buttocks. Breathe comfortably as you "walk" forward in your seated position; bring your right foot forward and then your left, creating a forward motion. Be careful that your baby's legs don't fall between your thighs; if this is happening, hold your baby under the buttocks. Keep breathing. Keep your chest open and your back tall. Now reverse direction to go backward.

If you are doing this without your baby, use your arms to help with the back-and-forth motion.

Body check: Use your abdominal muscles and squeeze your buttocks together. Lift up through your pelvic floor, keeping your chest open and bringing your shoulder blades on top of your ribs.

Baby check: Make sure Baby is having fun. I like to sing the "Ants Go Marching" song while I go visiting!

Repetitions: Ten steps forward, ten steps backward

Lie down on your back.

Pelvic Tilts

Do three pelvic tilts with your baby resting against your thighs. She'll enjoy the ride!

Knees-to-Chest Rocker

Rock back and forth and side to side as many times as you like.

Rock up into a seated position.

Leg Lifts with Baby

Do three leg lifts.

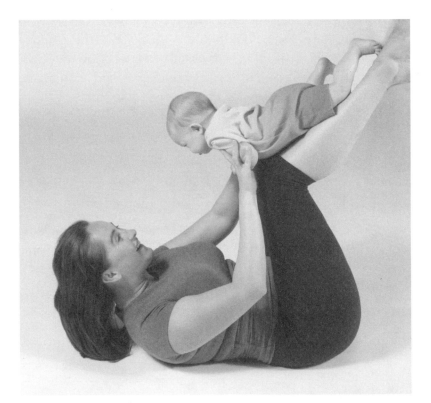

Forward Bend with Baby

Hold this bend for three breaths.

Half Spinal Twist

Hold the twist for three breaths on each side.

Upper Back-Chest Stretch

Another one of my favorite stretches, this is great to do for an achy upper back. If you feel as though you've been breast-feeding all day, try this.

Where's Baby: In front of you or on your lap.

To begin: Seated in a cross-legged position, raise a strap over your head. Your arms should be comfortably apart. Inhale, exhale and lower the belt behind your back, staying at the place where you feel a lovely stretch through your chest and upper back. Take three breaths, then lift up the strap and bring it down to the front.

Body check: Ground your sits bones and lengthen through your spine so you are not slouching.

Repetitions: Hold at least once for three breaths and repeat as many times as you like.

Move into the final relaxation pose.

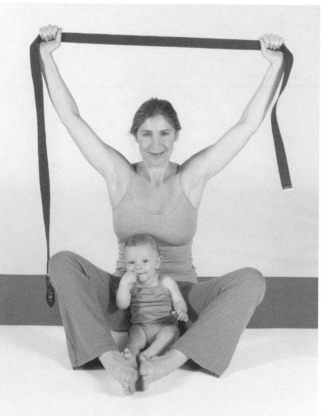

Supported Reclining Pose

This very calming position opens up the chest and helps respiration.

Where's Baby: On a blanket beside you or resting on your belly or chest

Props: Cushion, pillow or blanket

To begin: Lie down on your back on the floor or a bed. Place a cushion between your support and your back, under your chest area and parallel to your spine. Position your head and chest slightly higher than your abdomen, pelvis and legs. Roll two blankets up and put them under your knees. Let your arms extend away from you, palms facing the sky.

Body check: Make any adjustments to your position so that you are comfortable.

Length: As long as you want

> ⇥ **ROUTINE 4 (APPROXIMATELY 50 MINUTES)** ⇤

Begin in a seated position (cross-legged if it is comfortable for you), with your baby next to you or on your lap.

Forward Neck Release

Do three of these.

Extend your legs forward.

Foot Stretch

Make sure you stretch each foot for at least a minute and rotate it at least five times in each direction.

Come onto your hands and knees.

Child's Pose

Hold this for three breaths; it's a good pose during which to practice your kegels.

Stand up slowly by opening your feet a little wider, bending your knees and walking your hands toward your knees to come into an upright position. Slowly stand.

Sun Salutation (Soorya Namaskaram)

This series of postures flows gently from one into the next. The sun salutation is best done in the morning; it's also a great warm-up exercise that will keep the body flexible. Begin with one round and progressively add more.

Where's Baby: Lying in front of you. Make her part of the sun salutation as you wiggle your fingers at her, smile at her, kiss her.

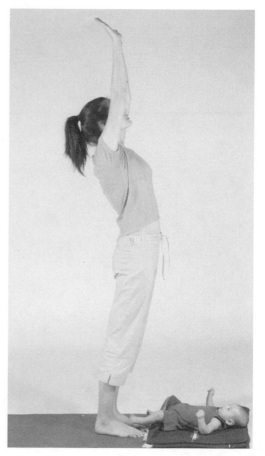

1. Stand tall, with your feet about one inch apart and your arms alongside your body. Check your posture. (This is actually a pose called *tadasana,* or "mountain pose.")
2. Bring your hands into prayer position. Inhale, stretching your arms up alongside your ears. Bend back gently; use your abdominal muscles and squeeze your buttocks to protect your lower back.
3. Exhale and hinge forward, lengthening through your spine and allowing your torso to hang over your legs.
4. Bend your knees. If your baby is in front of you do a few bicycles with his legs and say hi to him. Now bring your fingers in line with your toes.

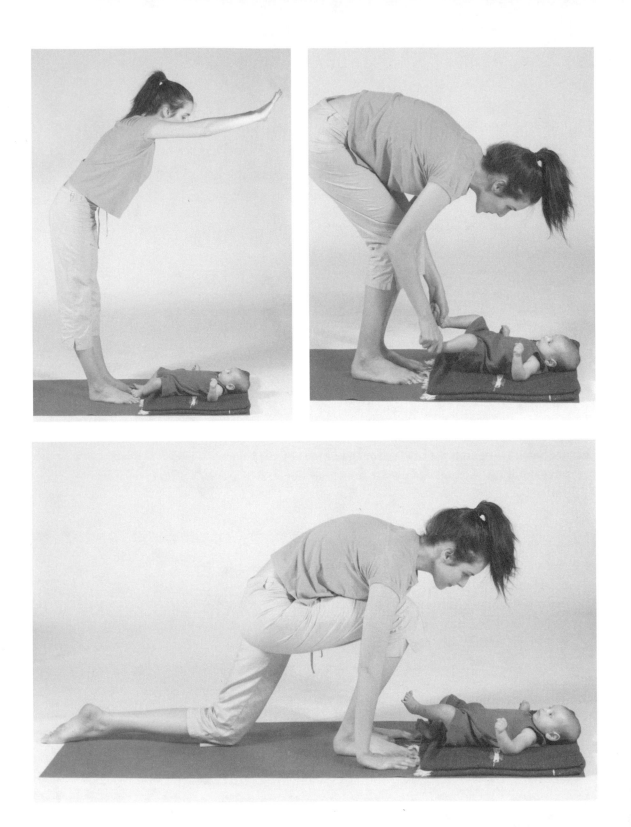

5. Stretch your left leg back, bringing your left knee to the floor. Inhale, raising your arms over your head and gently looking up.

6. Exhale, lower your arms back to the floor, and stretch your right leg back, coming into downward dog.

7. Lower your knees, chest and chin to the floor, keeping the pelvis raised.

8. Lower your pelvis and come into cobra. Make contact with your baby—do a couple raspberries, kiss his belly.

9. Curl your toes underneath. Exhale and come up to downward dog.

10. Bring your left leg forward and your right knee to the floor. Inhale, raising your arms over your head and gently looking up.

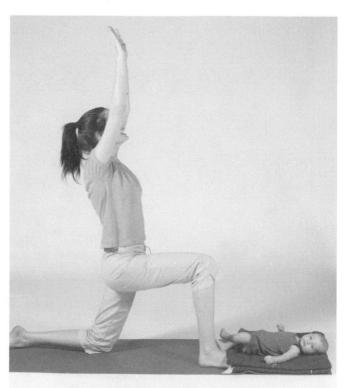

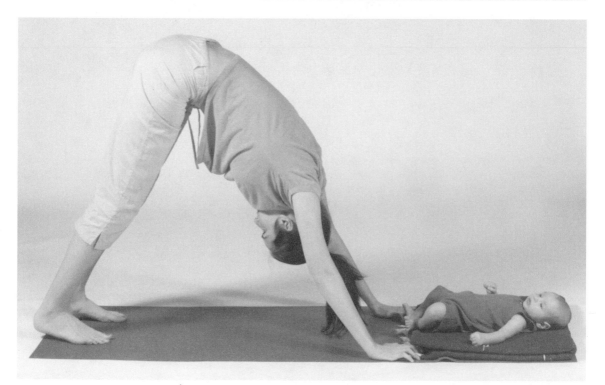

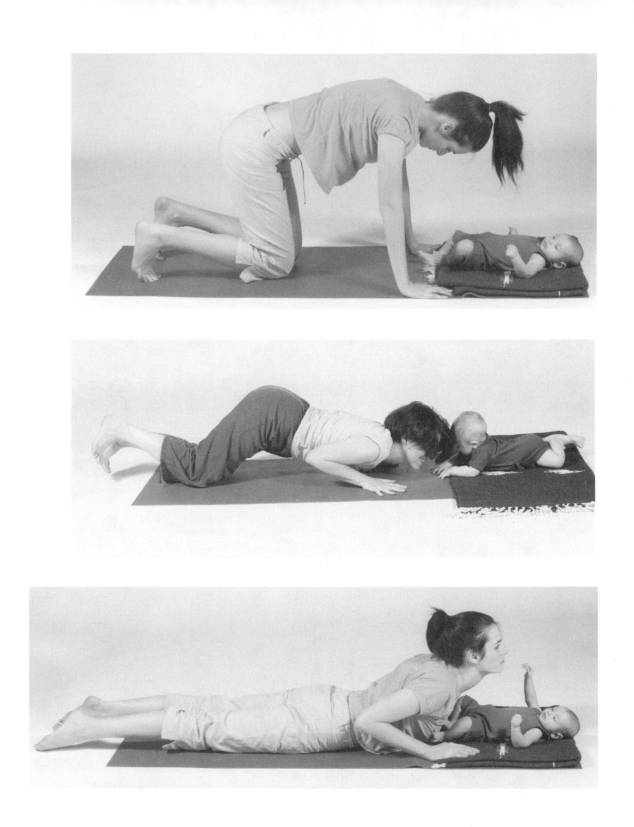

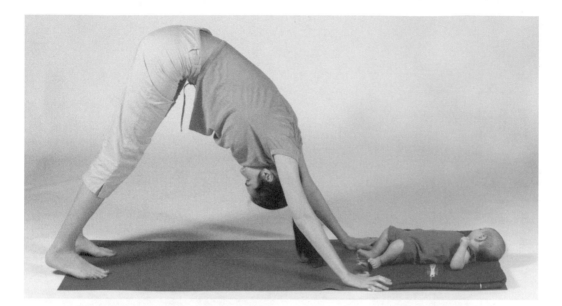

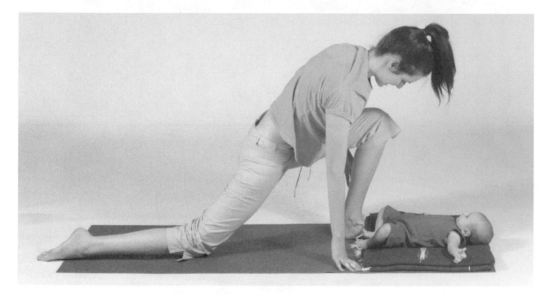

11. Exhale and bring your hands back to the floor, bringing your
    right leg forward and letting your torso hang over your legs.

12. Lengthen forward through the spine with your arms extended
    in front. Inhale and come up to standing with your arms
    alongside your ears. Gently bend back, using your abdominals
    and squeezing your buttocks.

13. Exhale and bring your arms down alongside your body to end
    in mountain pose.

Three Months to

One Year

215

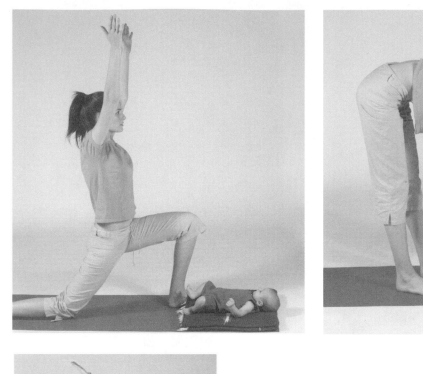

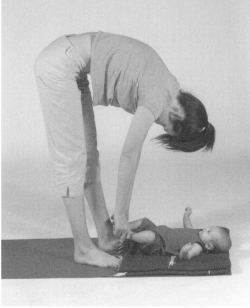

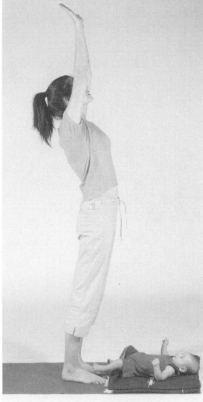

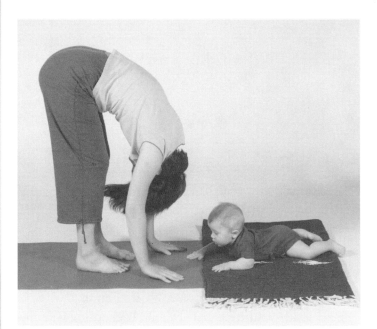

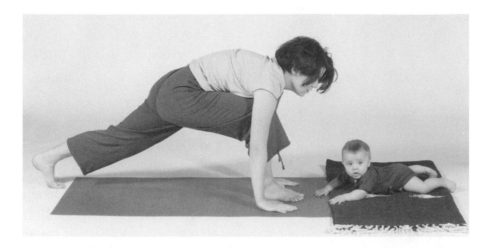

Advanced variations: In position 5, keep your left knee off the floor, and when you repeat this lunge on the opposite side in position 10, keep your right knee off the floor. You can also add the plank pose between positions 6 and 7.

Body check: Check your body alignment after each position.

Repetitions: For starters, do one round slowly. Work up to three rounds, then add more. Once the positions are learned, see if you can make them flow from one into the next. The sun salutation can become a meditative movement; I often do ten repetitions as my practice.

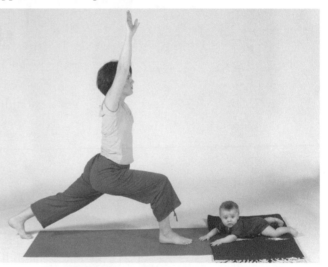

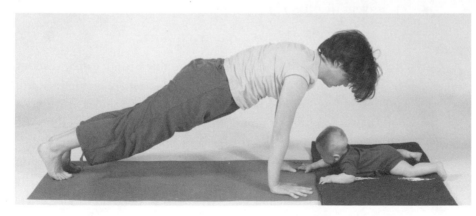

Uddiyana Bhanda and Variation

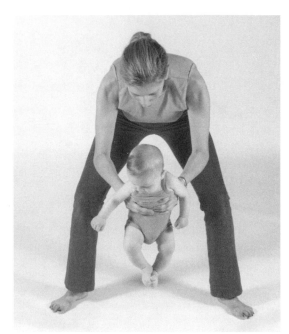

This pose works the abdominal muscles.

Where's Baby: On a blanket in front of you

To begin: Stand with your feet shoulder width apart. Inhale. As you exhale, bend forward and bring your hands just above your knees. Draw your abdomen in and up. As you slowly exhale all the breath out, keep lifting the belly up. Inhale, and come up to standing. Exhale, inhale and repeat.

Variation with Baby: Holding your baby around her ribs, inhale, exhale, bend your knees. Lift your belly button up toward your spine. Swing your baby gently back and forth and come up to standing.

Repetitions: Three times

Triangle

One of my favorite poses, triangle strengthens the legs and buttocks, increases flexibility in the spine, stretches side muscles and opens your rib cage, hips and chest.

Where's Baby: On a blanket in front of you

To begin: Stand with your feet a comfortable distance apart (about the length of one leg). Your feet, hips and chest are facing forward; you're standing tall and using your abdominal muscles. Turn your right foot in on a slight angle; then turn your left foot to the side. Lift your arms up parallel to the floor and even with your shoulders. Inhale, exhale and stretch to the left side. Inhale, raising your right arm. Exhale and reach your left arm down to your left leg. Advanced yogimamas can bend their left knee, bringing their left elbow to knee. Cross your right arm behind your back; your left arm goes underneath your left leg to grasp your right hand. Hold for three breaths. Inhale your body back to center. Switch your foot position and repeat to the right side.

Body check: This posture can be practiced against a wall for support. It's important to feel a good stretch to your side muscles; it does not matter how far down the leg you come.

Repetitions: Hold for twenty breaths on each side.

Come back to the floor by going into a squat or bringing one knee down and then the other. Turn onto your belly.

Cobra

Hold this for three breaths.

Roll onto your back.

Pelvic Tilts

Do three pelvic tilts, with your baby coming along for the ride.

The Bridge

The bridge works the buttocks (gluteus muscle), which helps alleviate stress on the lower back. It also stretches the fronts of the thighs.

Where's Baby: On your thighs or on a blanket in front of you

To begin: Lie on your back and bend your knees, keeping the soles of your feet on the floor. Bring your belly button back toward your spine, squeeze your buttocks and raise your hips off the floor (or bed). In addition to the buttocks, also lift up and contract your pelvic floor muscles. If your baby is next to you, bring your arms underneath yourself, interlacing your fingers. Hold this bridge pose for as long as it feels good. To come down, bring your hands to your sides (unless you are holding your baby) and lower down ver- tebra by vertebra, bringing your pelvis to the floor.

If you are holding your baby on your thighs, you can also add bouncing up and down while singing "Bumping Up and Down" (see page 154). As you come into the bridge pose with your baby on your thighs, make sure to contract your abdominal, gluteus and pelvic floor muscles. Drop your hip to the right and left as you sing.

Body check: Use your abdominals and glutes.

Repetitions: Do once.

Advanced variation: Advanced yogimamas can push up to the wheel, as illustrated. This very energizing pose is a great backward bend. Bring your palms beside your ears with your fingers pointed toward your toes. Push up into wheel. To come out of wheel, bend you elbows and lower to the crown of your head. Slowing roll the back of your head down to the floor and then roll down vertebra by vertebra.

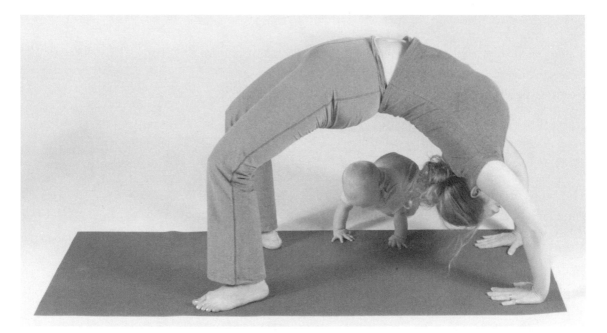

Now we're going to focus on the abs.

Abdominal Work I

This exercise tones and strengthens the abdominal muscles. You can do it on the floor or in bed.

Where's Baby: Resting against your thigh or lying next to you

To begin: Lie down on your back. Bend your knees, keeping the soles of your feet on the floor. Cross your arms over your midsection and exhale. Contract your abdominals by bringing the belly button back to the spine. Your chin moves toward your chest. Lower yourself back down again.

Body check: While doing this movement, it is important to focus on the abs; visualize them working. Do not use your neck or other muscles to raise or lower yourself.

Repetitions: Begin with five and work up to fifteen to twenty or whatever is comfortable per day.

Boat Pose (Navasana)

The boat pose tones and strengthens abdominal and thigh muscles. It's a good balance for the bridge pose. This is an advanced pose. For beginners, lift your legs and support your toes on a wall.

Where's Baby: Either on your lap, facing toward you so she rests on your thighs as you do this pose, or next to you

To begin: Start with your knees bent, feet flat on the floor. Balance on your sits bones. Slowly begin to stretch out your legs and lift them up. Keep balancing on the sits bones. First start with your hands on the floor, but work to lengthening your arms straight out parallel to the floor with your palms facing

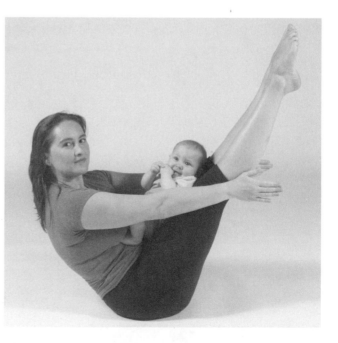

each other. Squeeze your inner thighs together. Keep lifting your breastbone. Hold for six to ten breaths.

Body check: Try to stay forward on your sits bones to keep your balance. At first you may feel wobbly, but keep trying. Keep your chest open so your back doesn't round. Smile at your baby!

Repetitions: Hold for six to ten breaths.

Abdominal Work III

These "crunches" strengthen your abdominal muscles. As you do these, visualize your ribs moving toward the pelvis.

Where's Baby: Resting against your thighs, with you using one or both of your hands to support her. As you lift your head and upper back, smile for her and play a game of peekaboo as you come up!

To begin: Lie on the floor (or a bed), your knees bent, the soles of your feet on the floor. Put your hands under your head. Exhale and contract your abdominal muscles as you lift your head and shoulders off the floor. Make sure to keep your elbows open out to the side and look up to the ceiling. Inhale, slowly lower your back down to the floor, keeping your abdominals engaged.

Body check: Make sure you keep your abdominal muscles engaged; don't use your neck muscles or hip flexors to help you.

Repetitions: Five to ten times, working up to twenty

Knees-to-Chest Rocker

Rock three times from side to side and front to back.

Rock up to a seated position, then stretch your legs out in front of you.

Full Forward Bend

Hold this for three breaths.

Come back down onto your back.

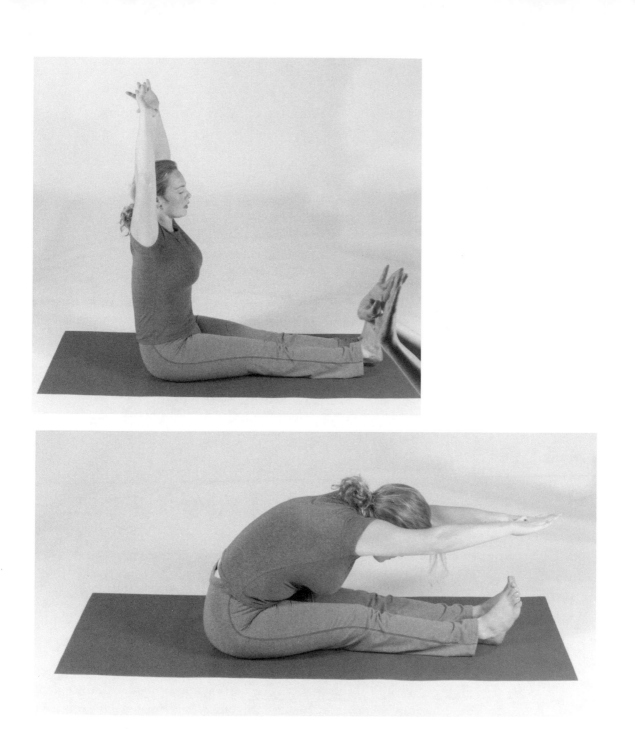

Knees-to-Chest Rocker

Rock again three times.

Baby Crocodile Spinal Twist

Twist to each side for three breaths.

Move into the final relaxation pose.

Savasana

Hold for as long as you like.

ROUTINE 5 (10–40 MINUTES)

Begin in a standing position.

Moon Salutation (Chandra Namaskaram)

Whereas the sun (Soorya) salutation is associated with the masculine, the moon (Chandra) salutation is associated with the feminine. This empowering series creates a feeling of alignment toward both the earth and heaven.

Where's Baby: On a blanket in front of you

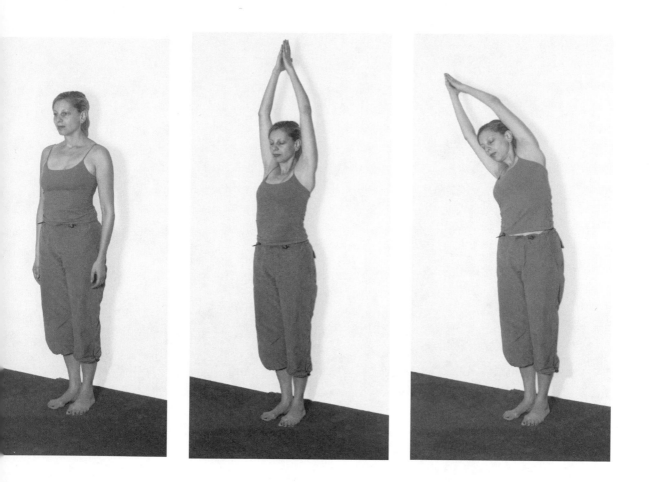

To begin:

1. Stand with your feet about one inch apart in "tadasana," (standing position or mountain pose); bring the toes in line with each other. Bring your hands into prayer position.

2. Inhale and bring your hands overhead.

3. Exhale and lengthen arms to the right in a side bend. Inhale back to center. Exhale, then lengthen arms to your left in a side bend. Inhale back to center.

4. Jump or step into a five-pointed star, with your arms outstretched. Stand with legs a comfortable distance apart.

5. Bring yourself into a goddess pose by bending your knees and elbows so your hands point up to the sky.

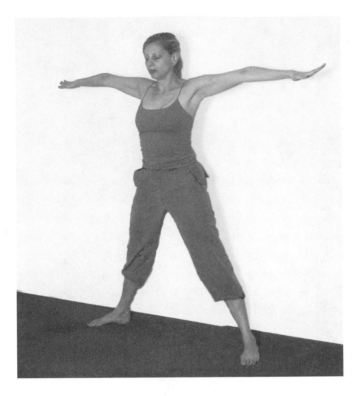

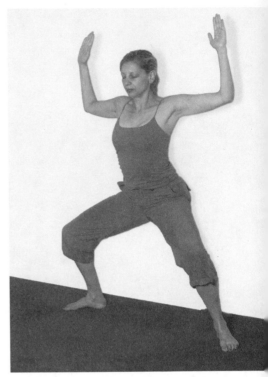

6. Straighten back into the five-pointed star.

7. Come into a triangle toward the right side.

8. Transition into a flying moon by resting your right palm on the floor or a block, lifting your left leg up, raising your left arm to reach up to the sky so you are balanced on your right leg and hand. Keep your left hip open. Stay here for a few breaths.

9. Bring yourself back to center, and repeat triangle and a flying moon on the left side.

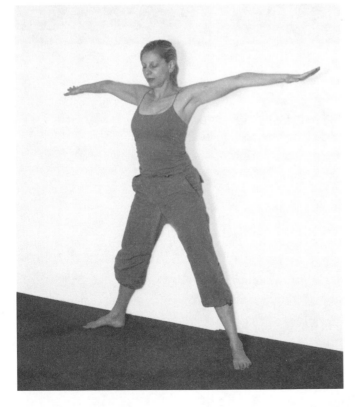

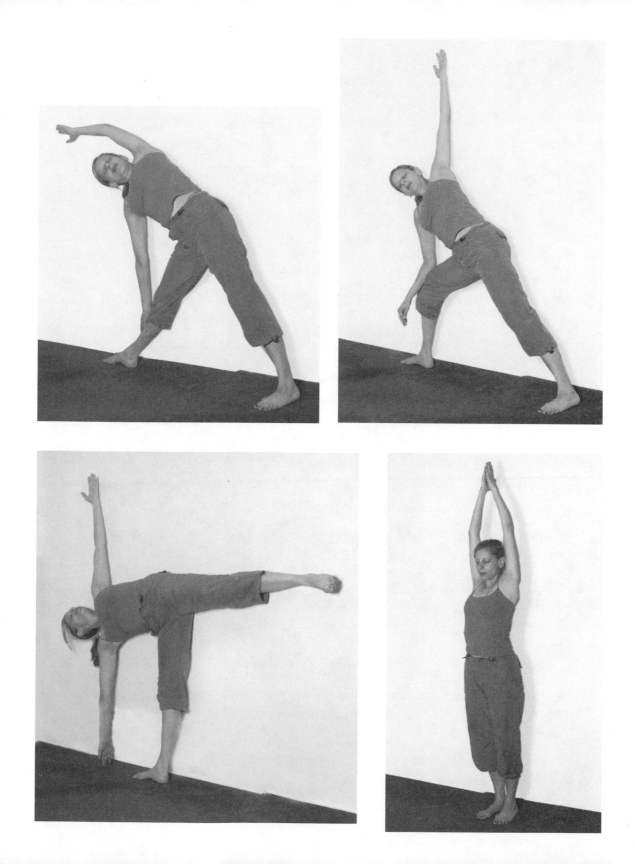

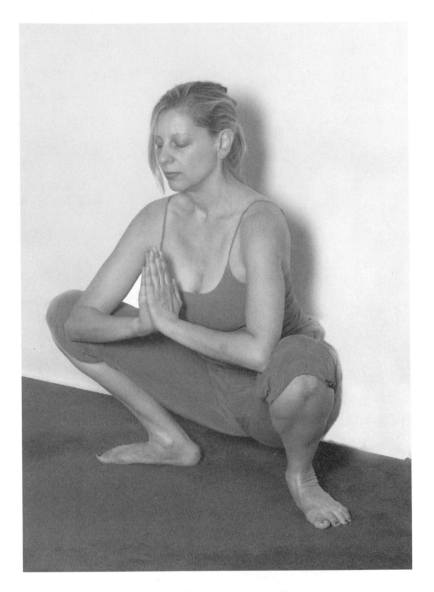

10. Come into a squat. Hold for three breaths.

11. Bring yourself back up into the five-pointed star.

12. Bring yourself into a goddess pose by bending your knees and elbows so your hands point up to the sky.

13. Come back into the five-pointed star, then jump or step legs together.

14. Raise your arms overhead, reaching to the sky, and lengthen arms to your left in a side bend.

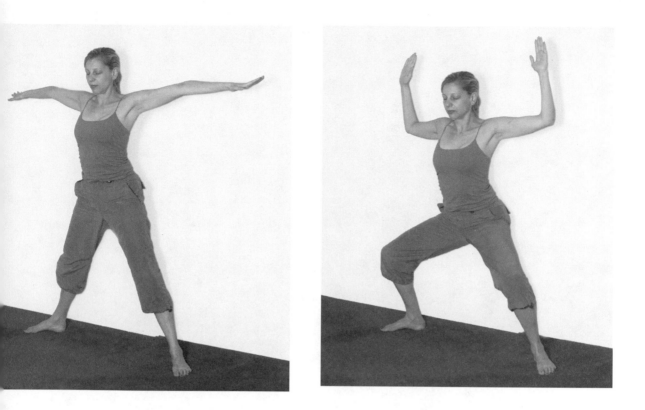

15. Bring yourself back to center. Side bend to your right. Come back to center.

16. Bring hands into prayer position, your feet one inch apart. Return to tadasana (standing position).

Repetitions: Do one round.

Supported Reclining Pose

Hold this for as long as you like.

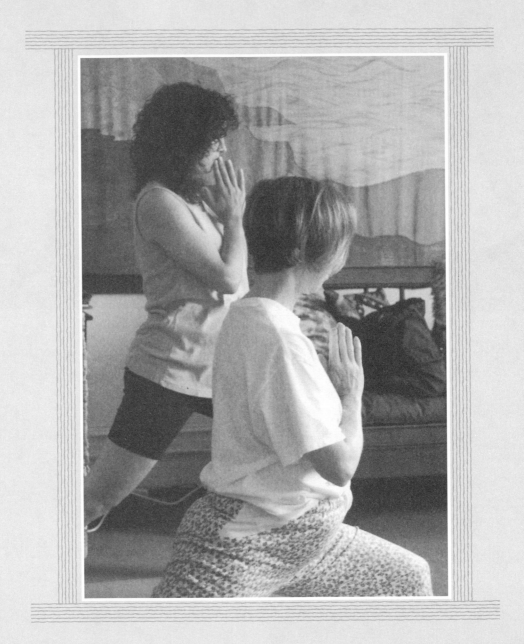

Eleven

Focused Routines

I've included these focused routines for those times when you want to relax (before and after having your baby) and when you wake up in the morning, plus a shortened routine for when you have only ten minutes. I know how busy and stressful motherhood can be! So I hope you will also be able to work these routines into your yoga practice.

Rainbow Stretch (for Prenatal and Postpartum)

If you have only limited time but need some peace of mind, try this terrific pose. It stretches the back, releases tension and relieves shoulder aches.

As you do your rainbow stretch, close your eyes and visualize different colors of light surrounding you and your baby. You can associate different colors with thoughts, such as pink for love, orange for life, blue for peace and so on.

Where's Baby: In front of you

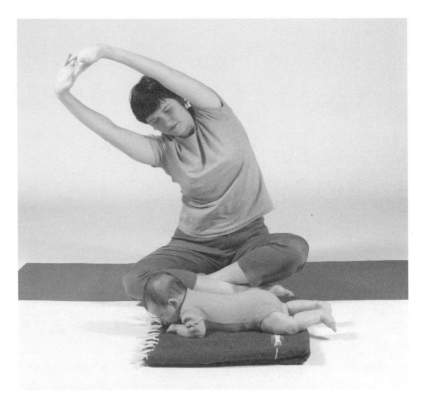

To begin: Sit in a cross-legged position or with your legs out in front of you, whichever is most comfortable for you. Press your sits bones down into the floor. Interlace your fingers and stretch your arms out in front of you, pushing your palms away from your body. Then bring your arms, fingers still interlaced, over your head. Trace big circles in the air with your hands and arms. Keep your sits bones grounded. Lengthen up through the spine and breathe as you do these.

Body check: Be aware of how your ribs feel and give them a nice stretch. Remember to breathe!

Repetition: Do three circles in one direction and then switch.

This is a great series to do after you have put your baby to bed or down for a nap, or anytime you need some tension relief.

Begin in a seated position.

Half Neck Rolls

Half neck rolls relieve tension in the neck and shoulders. Do them slowly, with one breath flowing into the next. Be aware of what you are feeling in your neck and shoulders. Do three times on each side.

Rainbow Stretch

This movement stretches the back, releases tension and relieves shoulder aches. As you do three circles in each direction, close your eyes.

Forward Neck Release

This movement releases tension in your neck, shoulders and upper back. It also provides a nice stretch for the vertebrae in the cervical spine. Do this sequence twice.

Come onto your hands and knees.

Wag the Tail

This posture gives a good stretch to the muscles between the ribs. Wag your tail three times on each side.

Child's Pose

Child's pose provides a great stretch for the spine, in addition to relaxing your entire body and mind. It's a good position in which to practice kegels. Stay here as long as you like.

Reclining Pose

This very calming position opens up the chest and helps respiration.

Props: Cushion, pillow or blanket

For prenatal: Sit on the floor with a blanket, rug or mat underneath you, and gently lower yourself down to a position lying on your side, your knees bent. Place a blanket or cushion underneath your head and put a blanket or cushion between your knees. Take another cushion or folded blanket and rest your arm on top of it. Close your eyes and relax into the position, letting tension seep out of your body. Get to a place where you can let go, feeling as though there is no part of your body that you need to hold on to. With each exhalation, allow yourself to melt into the floor a little deeper.

For postpartum: Lie down on the floor or a bed on your back. Place a cushion between your support and your back, under your chest area and parallel to your spine. Position your head and chest slightly higher than your abdomen, pelvis and legs. Roll two blankets up and put them under your knees. Let your arms extend away from you, palms facing the sky.

Body check: Make any adjustments to your position so that you are comfortable.

Length: Five minutes at least, giving yourself more time if you can

Here's a quick yoga practice for when you have just ten minutes to spare. This series will make you feel good!

Medical caution: This routine is for postpartum only; do not do if you are pregnant.

Begin in a seated position.

Half Neck Rolls

Start with three half neck rolls to each side to relieve tension in the neck and shoulders. Do them slowly, with one breath flowing into the next. Be aware of what you are feeling in your neck and shoulders. Your baby can either be in your arms or lying next to you.

Shoulder Rolls

Do three shoulder roll circles in each direction to open up the chest and upper back and relieve tension in the shoulders. This posture helps moms who hold their baby in a front carrier, especially as he gets heavier. Do these whenever you need to!

Where's Baby: Your baby is next to you or in your lap.

Come onto your hands and knees.

Downward Dog

This is a terrific stretching movement for the back and hamstrings. It also strengthens the upper body and tones your abdominals. Your baby lies in front of you as you hold this pose for at least five breaths.

Come onto all fours.

Child's Pose

Relax into child's pose. When you come down, wiggle your head to tickle your baby with your hair or give her a "raspberry" on her belly.

Come up to a sitting position.

Half Forward Bend (Janusirasana)

This posture stretches and strengthens the back and hamstrings. Hold for five breaths. Your baby is on a blanket in front of you or in your arms.

Repetitions: Hold each side for twenty breaths.

Lie on your back.

Baby Crocodile Spinal Twist

This posture opens the chest and hips and gently stretches your spine. Your baby is on a blanket in front of you. Hold to each side as long as you like.

Savasana

This posture helps bring deep relaxation to your entire body while quieting the mind. Relax for five minutes.

Designed for postpartum women beginning at three months, this series wakes you up! It gets you moving in the morning, using all your body parts, and brings in fresh energy. This series is particularly nice to do after your baby's first feeding of the day.

Begin in a seated position.

Half Neck Rolls

Half neck rolls relieve tension in the neck and shoulders. Do neck rolls slowly, with one breath flowing into the next. Be aware of what you are feeling in your neck and shoulders. Do twice on each side. Your baby can either be in your arms or lying next to you.

Shoulder Rolls

Do three shoulder roll circles in each direction to open up the chest and upper back and relieve tension in the shoulders. Your baby is next to you or in your lap.

Come onto your hands and knees.

Child's Pose

Relax into child's pose, a great stretch for the spine.

Where's Baby: Your baby is lying in front of you. Hold as long as you like; it's a good position in which to practice your kegels.

From your hands and knees, come onto your knees. Bring one foot to the floor. Curl back toes underneath. Push off from the floor. You're standing!

Sun Salutation (Soorya Namaskaram)

Please refer to the sun salutation series on pages 211–217. These postures will flow gently from one into the next. Your baby is lying in front of you. Make her part of the sun salutation as you wiggle your fingers at her, smile at her, kiss her. Do three rounds slowly.

Lie down on your back.

Shoulder Stand (Sarvangasana)

This posture tones the buttocks, lengthens the spine and improves balance. It also helps with digestive problems. Do not do shoulder stands if you are menstruating or have neck or eye problems. Your baby is on a blanket in front of you. Hold your shoulder stand for two minutes.

Fish Pose

Please do this pose to complement shoulder stand. Fish stretches the thyroid gland in the opposite direction. Hold for at least three breaths.

Come up to a sitting position, with your baby next to you or sitting with you.

Half Spinal Twist (Ardha Matsyendrasana)

This pose does much more than tone the abdominal area—it also stretches the back and side muscles, helps with digestive problems, keeps the spine flexible, squeezes toxins out of the spine as if one is "wringing a washcloth", and massages internal organs. Hold for three breaths on each side.

Yoga Mudra

This position seals in the positive energy that you've created from the breathing and asanas you've completed. Do not do this pose if you have knee problems. Your baby is on a blanket in front of you. Relax into this posture for one minute.

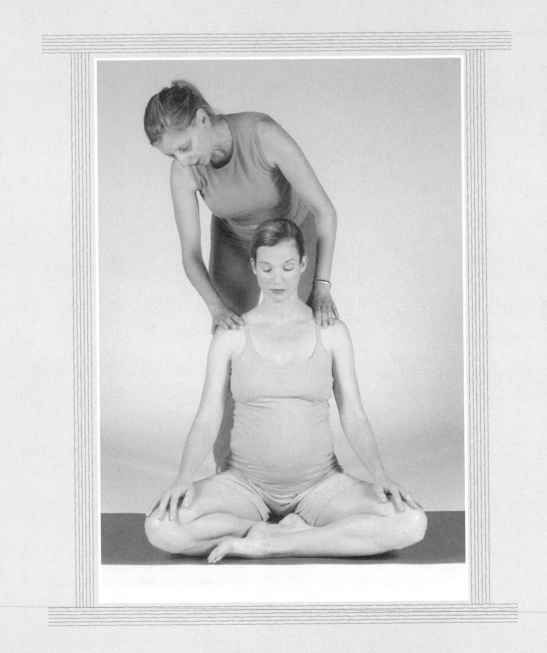

Twelve

Partner Postures

It can be a fun and different experience to include someone else in your and your baby's yoga. Give these poses a try with a partner or friend. Your partner will find a new way to bond with you and your baby, and your baby will discover and delight in the touch and attention of another person besides mom.

Prenatal Partner Postures

Squats

Squatting with Partner: Stand facing each other, an arm's length apart. Take hold of each other's wrists. Support each other as you slowly squat down to the floor. Pull back slightly to feel a nice stretch between your shoulder blades. To come back up, push your feet into the floor as you lift with your buttocks and legs.

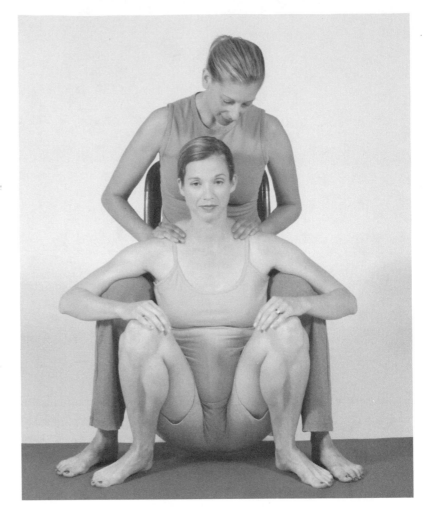

Labor Variation: Your partner sits on a chair and you sit between his legs, draping your arms over his legs for support. Your partner can give you a nice shoulder and back massage from this position.

Breathing Back to Back

Sit on the floor, back to back. Each of you can have your legs crossed or stretched out, whichever is more comfortable. Lean slightly into each other, keeping your backs lengthened and your

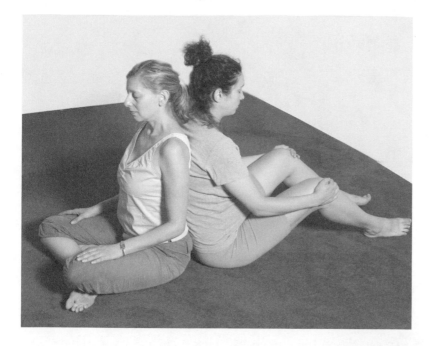

posture upright, and begin breathing. Concentrate not only on your breath, but on your partner's. Synchronize your breathing so that you are taking deep, long belly breaths and three-part breaths together. Feel each other's lungs expand and your bodies relax.

Right-Angle Stretch

Stand an arm's length away from a wall. Come into a right angle with the wall; extend to touch the wall as you flatten your back parallel to the floor and straighten your legs so they are parallel to the wall. Your partner places his hands at the top of your legs and gently pulls your pelvis toward him, giving you a great stretch in the legs and back while lengthening your spine. This is also a nice stretch to do on your own. I do this several times a day.

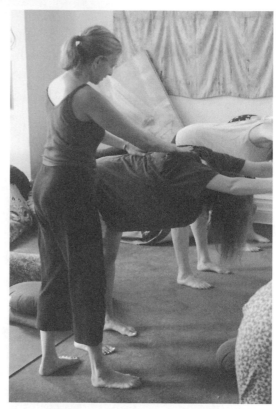

After-Birth Partner Postures

Breathing Back to Back with Baby

This is similar to the prenatal partner breathing, but now you will take turns holding your baby, transmitting energy to your child as well as your partner. Feel free to follow up with a round of oms.

Where's Baby: In the arms of one parent

To begin: Sit on the floor, back to back. Each of you can have your legs crossed or stretched out, whichever is more comfortable. One adult takes the baby into his lap, cradling the baby and letting her rest against his belly to feel his breath. Lean slightly into each other, keeping your backs straight and your posture upright, and begin breathing. Concentrate not only on your breath, but on

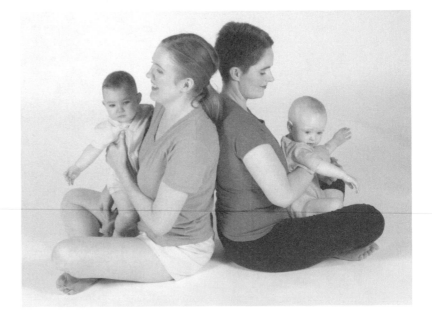

Yoga Mom,
Buddha Baby

your partner's. Synchronize your breaths so that you are taking deep, long belly breaths and three-part breaths together. Feel each other's lungs expand and your bodies relax.

Open V Stretch

This gives a nice stretch to the entire spine and the inner thighs.

Where's Baby: Your baby is in between your legs on the floor.

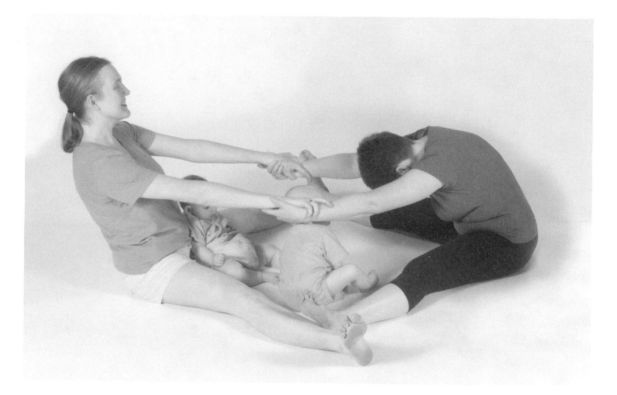

To begin: Sit on the floor with your legs in an open V position, your back straight. Your partner is facing you in the same position. Take hold of your partner's wrists and bring your partner forward over the baby. Stretch back and forth in a gentle movement.

Afterword

Yoga for a Lifetime

Moms tend to have a better understanding of
their bodies after giving birth. It wasn't until I
was pregnant that I realized how amazing the
body is, and all it can do. And it wasn't until
carrying Rachel as she grew and lifting a
stroller up and down subway stairs that I realized how important yoga is.

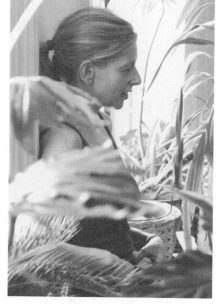

It continues to be important with the
next child: indeed, you need even more
strength managing a newborn along with a
young child. Yoga helped me keep up, physically and mentally, with the demands of
Rachel and Mikela.

You can continue to do yoga with your
kids for as long as they will let you. I remember
going to Rachel's preschool and doing
yoga with her entire class. After doing a few poses, I asked each
child to make up her own postures. I got a carrot pose and a radish
pose. Kids love to play, and you can incorporate yoga into playtime. You can do downward dog and tell the kids to go under the

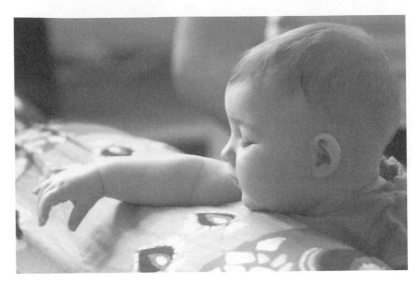

My baby and I both get a lot from the yoga; there's a give-and-take. We would do some mommy-focused yoga, then do something just for the baby, chanting or singing. There was time for me and time for her. And that was an incredible life lesson, this give-and-take. Maya's two now and she does her own yoga. She creates her own little downward dogs.

—VIRGINIA AND DAUGHTER MAYA

bridge you have made with your body. Mikela still loves when I do leg lifts with her on my shins.

And remember: kegel and abdominal exercises are important to do for the rest of your life, as are focused breathing and relaxation postures. Continue to work toward having a balanced mind, body and soul.

As you know, life will continue to present us with challenges, so continue to practice yoga. I don't know who said, "The days are long, the years go fast," but I do believe it. Enjoy your time with your baby. Before you know it he will be a toddler, school-age, then a teen (as I'm finding out!). Continue to grow in love, peace and joy as your baby does.

Jai (victory), amen, hallelujah.

Namaste,
Jyothi

Afterword

Index

Index

About the Authors

JYOTHI LARSON teaches hundreds of moms and babies prenatal and postpartum yoga at her popular mother and baby yoga classes, which she has been leading for ten years. She has studied yoga for more than twenty years and holds advanced teacher certification in hatha yoga from the Integral Yoga Institute in New York City. She also teaches at Healing Works, Soho Sanctuary, and Yoga People. Her two daughters, Rachel and Mikela, do beautiful sun salutes and downward-facing dogs.

KEN HOWARD is a journalist who writes about science, medicine and technology. He has been practicing yoga for ten years.